THE *Last*
CHOCOLATE
BROWNIE

THE *Last* CHOCOLATE BROWNIE

DAVE COURTEEN

authorHOUSE®

AuthorHouse™
1663 Liberty Drive
Bloomington, IN 47403
www.authorhouse.com
Phone: 1-800-839-8640

Published by AuthorHouse   06/26/2012

ISBN: 978-1-4685-7775-4 (sc)
ISBN: 978-1-4685-7776-1 (e)

Dave Courteen will donate all of his proceeds from the sale of this book equally between the following two charities:

The Woolverstone Wish Appeal which operates under the NHS Ipswich Hospital Charitable Funds, a registered charity In England (Number 1048827). The Appeal raises funds to refurbish the chemotherapy outpatients clinics and day unit in the Woolverstone Wing of Ipswich Hospital where his wife received her treatment for breast cancer

Breakthrough Breast Cancer, a registered charity in England (Number 1062636) and Scotland (Number SC039058), to help realise the charity's vision of a future free from the fear of breast cancer.

This book is Dave's personal account of his wife's experience of breast cancer and the opinions and statements it contains reflect his perspective and experience. They should not be regarded as a statement of current medical knowledge about the nature and treatment of breast cancer or of Breakthrough Breast Cancer's views and policies.

For information about breast cancer and breast awareness please see Breakthrough Breast Cancer's website, www.breakthrough.org.uk.

FOR MIRANDA

May you experience this vast, expansive, infinite,
indestructible love that has been yours all along.
May you discover that this love is as wide as the sky and as
small as the cracks in your heart no one else knows about.
And may you know, deep in your bones, that love wins.

Quoted from "*Love Wins*" by Rob Bell

CONTENTS

PHASE ONE—THE CHEMOTHERAPY

PHASE TWO—THE MASTECTOMY

PHASE THREE—THE RADIOTHERAPY

PHASE FOUR—MOVING ON

ACKNOWLEDGEMENTS

The virtual word of the web never ceases to amaze me. I started writing a blog and suddenly found that it acquired followers with whom I had no previous contact and from all four corners of the globe. As our story unfolded, the comments and messages these followers sent provided a vital source of support and encouragement to us, especially when the going was a tough. To everyone who followed the blog or left a comment I want to thank you so much. We valued so much that you joined us on our journey.

The idea of collating my posts into a book first came from my cousin, Kris Saunders, who remained an avid and loyal follower of the blog. There have been numerous others who encouraged me to make this into a book and helped me along the way. It has been more fun than I could have imagined. Thank you for inspiring me to make this project happen. I would also like to thank the team at AuthorHouse who have led me through the publishing process.

Clearly the main impetus for this book has been to raise funds for Breakthrough Breast Cancer and I want to thank the team at their head office for all their support in marketing and promoting the book. I really hope that this book generates revenue that will support the vital work they do.

I am also raising funds for the Woolverstone Wish Appeal at NHS Ipswich Hospital with the aim of helping to improve the facilities within the oncology department where Miranda received her treatment. Miranda and I are hugely grateful for the incredible care and attention that she got from the medical profession during her illness. I would like to particularly record our thanks to the nursing teams within the Woolverstone Wing of NHS Ipswich Hospital where Miranda received her chemotherapy and radiotherapy treatments and to the staff at the Nuffield Hospital in Ipswich where Miranda had her mastectomy. Their compassion and care was exceptional.

I would particularly like to acknowledge the guidance and support of some of the leading professionals who managed Miranda's care. Jane Aitken became Miranda's consultant just prior to her mastectomy and her calm reassurance coupled with her skills as a surgeon provided us with much needed confidence at a critical time. Dr Liz Sherwin is Miranda's oncologist and we are so grateful that her chemo recipe was so successful. More than that though, throughout this process Dr Sherwin has been a constant source of reassurance and encouragement. We always felt that she had so much time for us despite the demands and pressures of the NHS system and we are very grateful that every question we asked, no matter how daft it may have been, was always given a full and detailed response. Finally the provision of Rachel Clifton as our MacMillan Breast Care Nurse Specialist was a vital lifeline for Miranda. Rachel has that happy knack of being in the right place at the right time, was always on the end of the phone when Miranda most needed her and made the whole treatment programme seem manageable even when we felt like we had a mountain to climb. Whatever money we raise to support their work will never repay the debt we owe for the support and treatment Miranda received.

We have been so blessed to have many friends who have been incredibly supportive throughout Miranda's illness and if you were one of those who sent us emails, texts or who phoned us or who helped practically with childcare or dropping meals around to save us cooking then thank you so much. You played a huge part in this journey and we are so grateful to you all.

Thank you to everyone at the Forge Community Church. We believe in the power of prayer and we will forever be thankful that we were part of such a loving and supportive Church while we went through this.

To my Mum and to Barbara and Andrew, Miranda's parents, I want to acknowledge the huge amount of love and help you have showered on us. We are lucky to have such wonderful parents.

My sister-in-law, Lou and her family of Ju, Chloe and Sophie were an amazing source of strength and helped us in so many ways. Lou has been an active promoter of the blog and the book and at times felt like my closest ally as we shared the same deep love for Miranda and the same sense of helplessness as events unfolded. I couldn't have wished for anyone better to walk with me.

To Miranda, this book is about you, your incredible strength, your faith, your determination and your love. Thank you for allowing me to write it and for sharing your own thoughts along the way. You have been an inspiration to so many people but I wonder if you will ever realise how much you have inspired me too. Thank you for showing me what it means to live out a life full of 1 Corinthians 13. I am so excited and grateful to be able to walk with you, by your side, forever.

And finally I want to thank my two daughters Rose and Millie. This is your story too. Thank you for the sense of fun, laughter and love you have both brought into my life. Of all the roles I have in life, being your Dad is by far the best. I hope that some time in the future, when you become adults, this story will help you understand what we all experienced and that you will realise just how blessed you are to have the Mum that you do. I'm sure you will. And may you be forever reminded that my love for you is immeasurable; that I am proud of you, not for anything you have, or will, achieve but just because you are my daughters.

1

The Journey Begins

Do you remember the film—Notting Hill? There's a group of friends all sat around the dinner table and telling their hard luck stories with the intention of winning the last remaining chocolate brownie.

Well this book, to a certain extent, is the hard luck story of my family but I hope that you will consider it also filled with humour, hope and encouragement. My story starts in early 2010 when my wife, Miranda, found a lump in her breast. After mammograms and MRI scans gave the all clear we heaved a sigh of relief and got on with life. However when she found another lump in her neck at the end of the summer she was referred for further checks and this included visits back to the breast clinic and the ear, nose and throat consultant and the haematologist for good measure! Initially all tests proved encouraging but a final third mammogram in November found that the growing tumour in her breast was in fact cancerous and we entered a whole new world. The cancer Miranda has is less common and has behaved abnormally. It's a type that doesn't always show up on MRI scans or mammograms. It also found its way into the lymph nodes in her neck and so began a journey into a life of uncertainty and chemotherapy.

Miranda started her treatment on Christmas Eve 2010, and, at that point in time was scheduled to have 18 weeks of chemo followed by surgery to remove part, or maybe all, of her breast and some of her lymph nodes in her neck and armpit. She was then to continue with chemo until December 2011.

The purpose of this book is to tell my story, of a worried husband, trying to be as supportive and encouraging as I can to my rather wonderful wife and our two daughters, Rose and Millie, who were 5 and 2 years old respectively and not really sure what was happening to our family. It started as a blog; a virtual diary. The blog somehow attracted a far wider following than I ever imagined and I was encouraged by numerous comments and suggestions to turn it into a book and so here it is!

So why did I start a blog? Well clearly there was a real cathartic benefit for me in committing my thoughts and feelings to "virtual paper". I also realised that for some of our friends it is really hard to know how to be supportive and I hoped the blog would provide anyone with the opportunity to post a message of support and encouragement. And they did, and Miranda and I really appreciated that. We also recognised that a blog is a good vehicle for updating people on the progress of treatment and saved us from making sure we had updated everyone individually of our latest news and developments. It also seems that some people found our story and journey with cancer helpful as they dealt with their own struggles that life inevitably delivers.

You will find the book tells the story just as the blog did, with diary style updates as Miranda's treatment programme evolved. We learnt very quickly that a journey with cancer can be a bit of a rollercoaster ride at times. But it was a journey that we started out on with hope in our hearts, prayers on our minds and an absolute fierce determination that there would be laughs along the way and a positive outcome. Maybe, at times, we'd feel like we earned the last chocolate brownie but maybe we should leave that for others to decide.

Thank you for taking the time to read our story and we hope you are pleased you shared our journey . . . .

PHASE ONE

THE CHEMOTHERAPY

2

In a Fog

So as I sit and write this—it's 1am in the morning and I've just driven Miranda to the hospital through thick fog as she has developed a fever and they are concerned she has developed neutropenia. This apparently is quite common with cancer patients receiving the same chemotherapy treatment as Miranda. It's not great as it basically means there is an infection attacking her body which her body can't fight off because of the lack of white blood cells that have been taken out by the chemo. If she's got this it will mean a few days in hospital on an intro-venous antibiotic drip.

Up until now all had been going well—Miranda seemed to have the side effects of the chemo under control and we have just enjoyed a really good Christmas but tonight (29th)—day 5 of chemo—has been different. In a lot of discomfort and with a temperature we followed the advice in our "instruction manual" and rang the hospital ward to explain the symptoms and next thing we know here we are. Thank goodness the fog stopped the "in-laws" from going home as they are able to look after the children.

So the hospital is heaving—apparently it is so bad they are turning ambulances away at the door—and a perfect opportunity to update the blog as I think we could be waiting a while for the one doctor on call covering the whole of Ipswich Hospital!

The thing that really strikes me with this horrible illness and its treatment is that there is so much to learn—I'm only half joking when I talk about an "instruction manual"—we have a blue folder with all the details of side effects and what to do and the chemo "recipe" is over a page of what pills and medicines Miranda needs to take and when. And half of them are just to help neutralise the side-effects of the chemotherapy treatment itself. It seems so surreal. It is a steep learning curve and I need to start climbing.

Eventually the doctor arrives—looking all of 19 years old really—which doesn't fill me with confidence if I'm honest. She informs us that Miranda will need a chest X-ray and we are whisked off to find a spare examination booth. This involves a trip in a lift and opening up an area of the hospital closed and alarmed overnight. That was exciting in its own right.

Now I need your opinion on something. You see I'm one side of the curtain and the Doctor and Miranda are the other with the Doc by the sounds of it giving Miranda a top to toe examination. I can clearly hear everything that is being said and when the Doc gets to her stomach and associated areas I hear Miranda say "be careful around there—it's a bit windy tonight". So be honest—was it wrong of me to laugh out loud?! Really? I mean she wasn't talking about the weather was she!

Anyway it transpires that Miranda's results suggest she is borderline neutropenic and so she is staying in overnight, until she can be seen by an oncologist in the morning. There are no beds on the cancer ward so we trip across to the other side of the hospital in search of a spare bed. Now I realise its difficult when the hospital is full but it seems a stunning decision to put someone who has no ability to fight infection in the pre admissions ward which is full of people with swine flu and various illnesses waiting to be admitted to the main wards! We arrive to a chorus of coughing and wheezing the like of which you would only expect to hear at a smokers convention. It 3:15am and I've lost any ability to fight this decision so with Miranda safely "checked in" I head for home.

As I walk across the hospital car park I actually catch the first cries of the dawn chorus and have to admit that I have a "moment" as I realise the last time I experienced this dawn chorus in this very car park was when Millie was born. The difference in emotions and circumstances cuts through me like a biting cold wind on a frosty morning that leaves you fighting to catch your breath.

Its 4:30am and I'm home—fog safely negotiated and it's time for bed. In two hours my youngest will be demanding my attention and shortly afterwards both girls will be requiring an explanation as to why the Mum who safely tucked them up into bed last night has mysteriously disappeared to hospital while they slept.

You know that "journey" and that "road" I've talked about us travelling on—I think it might just be a bit hilly in parts. And tonight well I was in a real fog to be honest.

Goodnight!

3

What My Wife and Kylie Minogue Have in Common!

When Miranda was first diagnosed I spent a bit of time trying to find out about other people who had had the same disease and had beaten it. Just to see if there was anything we could learn from their experiences. So that's how I ended up reading about Kylie Minogue and her cancer story. One of the things that stuck in my mind was that she described her chemotherapy treatment as "like experiencing a nuclear bomb". Not overly encouraging that bit Kylie to be honest!

I had little perception of what chemotherapy would entail and the fact that Miranda just had to attend hospital for a few hours and not stay in overnight or anything when she received her chemo treatment seemed both manageable and fairly tame. Therefore having decided to write this blog I never expected that the first few would be written late at night whilst I was sat waiting for the "on call Doctor" at the hospital but once more that's where we are! It's Sunday night (2nd Jan) and Miranda has another temperature and a really nasty swollen face. So with a low blood count still as the chemo is doing its job we have no option but to head off to hospital to see if she is neutropenic and needs antibiotics more powerfully than can be given orally.

So let's just give you a real quick overview here—Miranda had her first dose of chemotherapy on Christmas Eve so we are 9 days in to a 21 day cycle before the next dose. We were led to believe that she would start to feel the effects of the chemo after a couple of days and that this would last for about a week before she would start to feel better. And when she felt just a few aches and pains after the first four days in I think we were both lulled into a sense that this was as bad as chemo got. We should be so lucky . . . . lucky, lucky, lucky as our friend Kylie might have said!

After 5 days she was in real pain and discomfort and our first trip to hospital on December 29th led to a two day stay before she was let home. The chemo has really kicked in now and she is completely wiped out, has a nasty rash, sore mouth, the works. To make matters worse her jaw has gone into spasm and this makes it difficult to open her mouth and to eat her food. So 9 days in and we're learning fast just how intense and harsh this chemo thing really is. I think that probably it will transpire that the chemo will leave her feeling pretty ropey for about 12/14 days of the 21 days between doses.

Anyway—back to tonight and since starting this we've seen the Doctor and the decision is that she needs to stay in hospital and that they think the swollen face is probably due to an infection rather than a muscle spasm. This means a dose of really strong antibiotics and that she'll be in hospital for at least 3 days and probably 5. That's a bit of a blow to be honest for Miranda and for all of us to be fair.

I think that we will take the next dose of chemo a lot more seriously and right now I'm sure my wife would whole-heartedly agree with Kylie's description of going through chemotherapy. So that's two things she got in common with Kylie then—their chemo experience and a cute bottom! Am I allowed to write that sort of thing? Oh well I have anyway, it's 3am and I'm beyond caring! These late nights are catching up with me!

4

Bring on the Tooth Fairy

It's great to be able to post some really positive news! I've just got back from visiting Miranda and she is on fine form—looking so much better. Her swollen face from the start of the week which had her feeling so awful and hardly able to eat has pretty much returned to normal. I no longer feel like I'm visiting a "cabbage patch" doll created in my wife's image—and that is her description of how she looked and definitely not mine I hasten to add!

It seems to have baffled a variety of specialists and consultants as to what has caused the problem with her face but as the antibiotics have taken effect they have been able to see into her mouth much better. The final conclusion seems to be that the problem is being caused by her wisdom tooth which came through bizarrely when Millie, our youngest daughter, was born. The tooth is gently rubbing on her cheek and normally this causes no problem but with no blood cells to fight any infection, the gentle grazing on the inside of her cheek, coupled with food remnants have caused a tiny infection which has gradually developed into the swollen face. Can't understand why she doesn't eat all her food. What a waste to leave some in her mouth!!

One of the things that I'm learning through this experience is just how much our bodies are doing all the time that we are just not aware of. Clearly we are constantly fighting off infection such as Miranda had without realising it. We really are wonderfully and creatively made.

The upshot of this infection for Miranda is that the wisdom tooth will have to come out and ideally before the next round of chemotherapy which is Friday week. It should be a simple process(!) and won't require a further stay in hospital.

So the plan is that Miranda will be out of hospital on Friday (7th) and will have a week to recoup and build up her energy before the next chemo a week later. To be honest I need to get her home as she has been having more "meetings" in hospital than I have been having at work such has been the number of visitors! And some of her visitors have been real troublemakers being told off by nursing staff for making too much noise and for sitting on the beds—a real hospital "no no" apparently!

But it has been great to hear the banter coming from the room when I arrive and to be able to sit with her and have some laughs and catch up just as we normally do at the end of the day.

Long may that continue! And of course when she gets home, minus her wisdom tooth, we can look forward to the tooth fairy visiting maybe! What is the going rate these days anybody know?

5

Surreal World

So today means Miranda is two weeks into her treatment and despite having a banging headache for most of the day she is feeling and looking a lot stronger. The next week will hopefully comprise plenty of rest and relaxing to build up her strength ready for round two of chemo next Friday. Obviously it's great to have her back home (that's an understatement as far as Rose and Millie are concerned!) and after all the "toing" and "froing" of the last fortnight it gives us both chance to pause and reflect a little on where we are.

To be honest it is all still a little bit surreal and although the events of the last week have brought a sharp realisation of what lies ahead, there are still moments when I find I'm metaphorically pinching myself to make sure this isn't all some kind of a weird dream.

I think there are three stages of acceptance that I've gone through in the month since Miranda was diagnosed. Initially there was just a numbness that I can't really explain or say that I've ever felt before. As we'd been to the breast cancer clinic twice before, and had experienced fairly long waits to see the specialist, I'd worked out that if a patient didn't reappear they had been diagnosed with cancer. Clearly they were taken back a different route so that they didn't have to walk through the waiting room, whereas those with the all clear came back through it. We'd always gone back through

14

the waiting room. So when we were told at the last visit that Miranda had cancer, bizarrely, the first thought that hit me was—we would be leaving the room by a different way. Random I know. I then remember trying to focus on what we were being told but finding it really hard to make my mind work.

The second stage for me was simply going through the upset and shock of the news. Miranda seemed to be much braver than me through this bit which is a bit pathetic of me I know!

After this, thank goodness, came a sense of determination to tackle this head on. I just felt that I can't influence what challenges or situations I face in life but I can determine how I deal with them, and this is something we all need to get on with. Of course, I can't pretend there aren't times when I get upset or when it all still seems so surreal, but I think I've got to a place where I've fully accepted the situation we, as a family, now face. And, of course, I am constantly reminded that however hard or tough this seems for me it is probably about a thousand times worse for Miranda. This is not the time for me to start living in the "feel sorry for myself" saloon.

So one month on from diagnosis what have I learnt?

Firstly I've learnt about the importance of accepting help from others. I'm normally the type of guy who likes to do everything himself in an "I need to prove I can do all this myself" kind of way so it has not been easy to allow friends in to help. But we've had no choice as I realise that we can't get through this on our own. So in the week leading up to Christmas when I needed to be at work, and Miranda was at the hospital every day for various tests, we had friends at home getting our ironing done, cleaning the house, wrapping Christmas presents and getting the wood in! Furthermore our freezer is now stocked to the hilt with meals kindly given to us by friends whilst Miranda was having her stays in hospital. We are so fortunate to have such great friends.

This help has been invaluable and we are of course so grateful—but I've learnt that by allowing others to help it has provided them with a way in to support us and feel involved. I think back to times when I've had friends facing challenging situations like we are now and I remember feeling helpless and not knowing how to provide support or show I cared. I think in this world in which we live it is easy sometimes to lose the sense of community and "everyone pulling together." When this is all behind us I'm determined to not lose the focus that in helping others in difficult times we gain so much ourselves. Although, thinking about it, I might need to draw the line at doing the ironing for someone as I'm just shocking at that particular chore—I seem to only be able to iron creases in not out!

I've also learnt that whilst we are determined to keep life as normal as possible we just have to redefine what is "normal life" for a while. We will live with this illness but not be ruled by it and we're certainly not allowing it to take over what we do. So that means that we can plan a little less, accept that for some periods of time Miranda may be popping into hospital at short notice, that my work schedule will get changed around a little so that I can be home for more bath and bedtimes for the girls. I may just have to catch up on work once they are asleep. I probably can't plan to be away overnight either. But that is it—otherwise everything else is the same and carries on as normal and we are all doing the things we were doing before. Rose is still at school, ballet and Rainbows, Miranda is still cooking, sorting the garden and playing the cello, I'm still working as much as ever, watching a bit of football, doing a bit of drama and drinking coffee(!) and Millie is still going to nursery and making us all laugh! So actually all pretty "normal" really and that is something we need to regularly remind ourselves of and be grateful for.

The third thing I've learnt is a growing realisation of what is important and what is not. It's a bit of a cliché but it is true—the most important things in life aren't things. There is no doubt that prior to this disease being diagnosed I took Miranda, and our girls, far too much for granted. I didn't afford them, and the time we spent together as a family, the attention or the focus they deserved. That's not to say that I didn't show them how much I love them or that we didn't spend time together—it was just that I didn't appreciate them and that part of my life like I do now. In addition there were things that occupied my mind and that I worried about that just didn't warrant the head space they took up and from now on I am determined to not let them back in. It is such a shame that it took this horrible disease to enter our lives for me to work that out.

As mentioned earlier I do a bit of drama at the Forge Community Church we attend. I love being part of that team and have some of the best times and biggest laughs with them during rehearsals. Every time we get to do the drama I get to read the part and I usually get to choose whether I want to play that role or not. It always amazes me that there are some roles that I read and immediately think to myself—yeah I could do that—and, of course, there are roles that I read and think the opposite and someone else takes the part. Life is about roles too. And generally we get to choose those roles—whether it is within relationships or through work—and I so love the roles that I get to play in real life. Of course, unlike the drama roles, life doesn't give us chance for a rehearsal—we just get the one shot at it.

However I didn't choose the role I now have to play supporting Miranda and the girls through this illness. If I'm honest, if I'd had the chance to "read the role" beforehand, I would have rejected it. It just wouldn't be me and it is not something I'm really suited to. I think that is why everything seems so surreal—I've been given a part and it doesn't feel like a fit. I can't work out why at this stage in our lives and those of our children we have to go through this . . . . but we do. So the other thing I've learnt over the past month is that just because we're given a role to play that we don't relish, we don't have to reject it, or get angry, or refuse to give it the same attention as other more suitable or enjoyable roles. It is by playing the most difficult and challenging roles that we learn and grow far more than when we are in a much easier role. So I'm accepting this role and am endeavouring to make it one of the most memorable and successful roles I've played.

Oh and finally one last thing—whilst I always knew that my wife is beautiful, full of fun, caring, compassionate and just a joy to hang around with, over the last month I've also learnt that she is brave, courageous, incredibly strong, determined and possesses an ability to trust in God which I'm still striving for.

And in this surreal world we are experiencing that has been a very reassuring and wonderful thing to discover.

6

This Much I Know
(Miranda's First Post)

Well after 5 posts from me we think it's high time you heard from Miranda! So her first "guest blog," written on the eve of her second dose of chemotherapy, gets straight to the heart of what it is like to have cancer.

It's very powerful and very honest so it comes with a "you might want a tissue when you read this" warning. I do love this girl so much . . . .

This much I know . . .

I know deep down that I should actually be getting on with cleaning the house now rather than sitting, spending / killing / wasting time, at the computer!

I also know that I'm a virgin blogger so please be gentle with me!

I also know that whilst I'm desperately trying so hard to feel positive today, it's really difficult to deal with handfuls of hair coming away when I washed my hair this morning. It's somehow worse than the thought of the next dose of chemotherapy tomorrow. That's something that nothing could have prepared me for.

I came away from the hospital last time with what seemed like pills for everything: steroids, anti-sickness, extra anti-sickness, pain relief, extra pain relief, laxatives, antibiotics, anti-fungals, anti-histamines, mouthwash, and creams for dry skin and a rash. That just about covered every eventuality and side effect, so I was well-prepared for the road that lay ahead! Or so we thought . . .

What we didn't fully appreciate (as you will know from Dave's blog) is how much infection your body fights against, without your knowledge, and when your immune system is low how susceptible your body is to any known or unknown weakness. And so the wisdom tooth was removed . . . the discomfort and frustration that came with not being able to open my jaw was not something the doctors could have prepared me for, and I didn't have a pill for it, and yet it was the one thing that got me down.

And now it's the hair loss. I have always known it was going to fall out, because that's something we all understand and accept as a side effect of chemotherapy. But that knowledge still doesn't quite prepare you for it. And it almost feels as though my identity is going to go with it—you have all, without exception, known me with long blonde hair, because I've never had the courage to do anything else with it! I'm just hoping it doesn't have the same affect on me as it did to Samson!

But, now I'm going to get all philosophical . . . I think it's the things for which you can't prepare yourself that grow you, strengthen you and you can surprise yourself how you cope when you come out the other side. Look at having children. The midwives can tell you all they know, but actually nothing will ever quite prepare a new parent for the shock of a) childbirth and b) holding this tiny little thing for the first time and the realisation that this little person is totally your responsibility and totally dependent on you, and you have not got a clue what to do with it! How scary is that?! But then don't we all surprise ourselves so often when we look at our children with such admiration and awe, and realise we're not really doing that bad a job, well, some of the time at least! And if I can find the strength to parent our children day-in day-out, when we have no idea what they are going to do or say next (I have a 2 year old!), then surely I can find the strength to face this treatment head on, as I have no idea what that is going to do to me next either!!

And so to courage. I keep being told how brave I am being at the moment, but I don't feel very brave, you know. I've just got to get on with it, as there is no other option. As we explained to our girls, it is the treatment and not the tumour that is going to make me feel unwell. That's a hard thing for me to get my head round, when I had been feeling fit and healthy up to Christmas Eve. But in accepting that, my focus is on the treatment and not the tumour, and I think that is how I am managing to deal with it. There is not a place in my mind which is entertaining any thoughts about what if the treatment doesn't work. Because there is no point going there, is there? There is no point contemplating what might happen. We'll deal with that if, or when, it arises. Life is carrying on as normal, it has to, for all our sakes, and we're just fitting in the treatment and the side effects around our everyday lives.

Those of you who cross paths with us regularly during the week will know that our lives are carrying on as they always have done. We still laugh lots, (we're finding new levels of black humour!), I still rant at my children, we're still the same people, and that's the best thing you have all done is to carry on being normal around us, because it's all the 'normalness' (yes, I know that's not a proper word but you know what I mean!) that makes life real for us! We might need a bit of help every now and again, and we're learning to swallow our pride and accept help—aren't friends and family just wonderful and amazing? We have been totally and completely overwhelmed *by all the support, help, love and prayers—we would have crumbled a long time ago if it was not for you!*

So just one final thought. I've accepted that I have no control over this. This illness. This treatment. The side effects. I don't really understand why this is happening. But what I have no control over, there is no point worrying about it, because there's nothing I can actually do about it. So I've decided to hand this all over to a being far greater than me, to God, and let him do the worrying for me, whilst I carry on merrily (most of the time!) going about my business and my life, and enjoying myself by spending quality time with my family and friends! And do you know, whatever you may personally believe, what an enormous weight has been lifted off my mind and shoulders! His shoulders are far broader than mine, and I'm fairly sure He can bear the load for me for a while.

Miranda x

7

Expect the Unexpected!

Part of the purpose of this blog is to help us update all of our friends that are spread around the country on Miranda's progress and so having had a dose of chemo yesterday I thought I would post a little "health update"

Expect the unexpected is the mantra that we are learning with this horrible disease. So having had a really smooth (if such a thing is possible) first chemo dose on Christmas Eve, yesterday's dose could not have been more different or more dramatic. But more of that in a moment—let's start with some excellent, positive news first!

Having been to see the consultant the first dose of chemo has been really effective and the tumour in Miranda's breast has significantly reduced while the lumps in her neck have all but disappeared. This shows that the chemo recipe they are using is working and is so encouraging. The reduction in the tumour is to such an extent that the consultant was considering putting a titanium marker in her breast yesterday so that when they get to the surgery in April they know for sure where the tumour was! However they have finally decided that, given the type of cancer that Miranda has, they are going to do a full mastectomy in May when the last round of chemo is finished and surgery can be safely carried out. Whilst, at 36, this is not the best piece of news for her, Miranda's is viewing this development as positively as ever and feels that by having a full mastectomy we can be reassured that they will have definitely removed all of the cancer whereas with a partial removal we may be left with the nagging doubt as to whether they have got it all.

So back to yesterdays chemo and after having the Herceptin, steroids and anti sickness drips fed into her as per normal Miranda was then connected up to the Taxotere. This drug is a really powerful chemical and as well as being responsible for the significant reduction in her tumour it has also been responsible for the nasty side effects including her rapid hair loss, neutropenia, etc. Despite the first dose going so well, this time as soon as the drug entered her bloodstream she immediately felt very unwell very quickly and experienced a kind of anaphylactic attack. She struggled to breathe, her vision became impaired and her face and chest went bright red. Suddenly nurses were appearing from every direction and various new drugs were put into her and after a very scary 5 minutes (seemed like an hour to me to be honest) Miranda felt OK again.

The end result is that they couldn't continue with the chemo and so we have to go back on Monday and go through the process again. As the Taxotere has been so effective, the medical team (and us) want to try again, only on Monday they will feed it into her more slowly and will administer antihistamine and hydrocortisone drugs as a pre-med drip. These are used purely to counteract a reaction to the Taxotere and by putting it in Miranda's system first they hope her body will tolerate it better than it did yesterday. If not then they will have to change the "chemotherapy cocktail" and use a different chemo drug, that is compatible with Herceptin, and we hope will work as effectively as the Taxotere is doing.

Once more we are reminded just how potent this treatment is and the "nuclear" power it possesses. So we have a little favour to ask. If you felt able to pray for Miranda that on Monday she could have the Taxotere drug administered safely, that Miranda's body tolerates it as well as it did on Christmas Eve and that it continues to attack the cancer as effectively, we would really, really appreciate it. We understand that some of you won't be comfortable doing this so maybe you could just think positive thoughts on Monday instead.

8

Hair Today . . . . Gone Tomorrow!

So you will know from Miranda's moving post that she is losing her hair and today we have been back to the wigmakers as she has changed her mind about her first choice wig—it's a women's prerogative apparently. The second (and final) choice is literally in the bag and we are now sat at the hospital for the second attempt at the second round of chemo—but that's a blog for another day!

Now understandably losing her hair has been one of the toughest things for Miranda to come to terms with. But the best way of dealing with it we have found is to maintain our sense of humour. So this post is written with Miranda's blessing and full support.

Her hair has, as we knew it would, disappeared very quickly; within a week to be precise. It's particularly noticeable at bedtime with tufts of it being left on the pillow. Indeed I have to be very careful if I sleep facing her, mouth wide open snoring. I find myself sucking in the hair and waking up making that horrible hacking noise that a cat makes when it has a fur-ball!

The visit to the wig shop was pure comedy gold. Tucked away on the first floor of a rickety building just off Ipswich High Street with the internals looking like they hadn't seen a paintbrush for a good couple of decades, it really was like a step back in time. When we walked into the shop itself I actually wondered for a moment if I was on the set of that 70⊠s sitcom "Are You Being Served". At any moment I expected Mrs Slocombe to appear talking about her pussy. (For those of you who are too young to remember this programme I'm not being rude this really was a part of the double entendre comedy). Of course as Miranda tried the various wigs on I was on top form with my favourite Eric and Ern "you can't see the join you know" quips.

Surprisingly Miranda actually said I was helpful and she valued my honesty and even agreed with me on the best choice. We were therefore able to leave with the assistant only mildly offended by my behaviour—quite a result to be honest. I knew she'd had enough of me when she left us to it and spent a good 20 minutes at the opposite end of the shop!

This really is just about the first time I've had anything to do with wigs although there was one famous occasion over twenty years ago when I worked at an up-market holiday centre in Lowestoft as the Sports Manager (now there's a rarity—the words "up-market" and "Lowestoft" appearing in the same sentence!). Anyway in the early and late season weeks we held "Over 50's" holidays which really translated as "Over 70's" to be honest. Hard as this will be to believe for those of you who know me but I used to take a "Popmobility" class. Very 80's I know but let me reassure you that I never wore leg warmers OK!

Clearly in the "over 50" weeks this "Popmobility" was fairly gentle exercise all done to Rod Stewart's "Maggie May" and Spandau Ballet's "True"—you get the idea. One week we had a very spritely old lady in her 80's with a full head of deep, red hair and who took part in everything we organised, including the said Popmobility class. I had all the participants doing a gentle sit up routine, on their backs with their hands on their thighs as they gently sat up. I can remember looking across the class and realising with horror that as everyone lifted their heads up this dear lady came up totally bald and left on the floor was this upside down red wig looking rather like a bird's nest that had fallen out of a tree! Stifling the urge to burst out laughing I got everyone to repeat the sit ups but this time with their hands firmly behind their heads!

Anyway I digress . . . .

So Miranda has a wig and to be honest it looks really good and I'd challenge anyone who saw her hair cut short to notice that in fact she has a wig. Indeed, to remain positive, we have now decided that there are some distinct benefits of a wig over natural hair and here are our top 7 benefits of wig wearing!:

1. It's cheaper—no need for expensive shampoos and conditioners or other hair products
2. It's easier to have a quick shower—and you don't need to wear a shower cap
3. It's quicker to get ready to go out—no straighteners or hair drying
4. You never wake up with a bed head or jimpy
5. When you go to the hairdresser (as you need to with a wig apparently) it is so much quicker. You can at least get on with the shopping and pop back in to collect it when it's been trimmed
6. When you're out you will never worry that you left the hair straighteners on
7. You can change styles in an instant—you just get another wig!

Every cloud has a silver lining! So there are our seven—over to you now. Can you think of any others?!

9

Like a Racehorse

This is just a quick post to let you know that the chemo treatment was completed successfully today and to thank you for all your positive thoughts and prayers.

It's been a long day and we are grateful to the nurses who worked so hard to make sure the drug was safely administered. It is fair to say that this is a pretty powerful drug and the day got off to a challenging start as, despite the smaller dose and having some counter-acting drugs first, the Taxotere still caused a reaction in Miranda when first administered. However, the reaction was much less severe and was controlled immediately as the nurses were on hand.

Eventually with the use of dilution by saline drip and a slower rate of dosing all the drug was administered by 6pm this evening—it took just under 6 hours to administer the same amount of the drug that was delivered in just over an hour the first time. But frankly, who cares! Miranda has had the drug she needs and we can move on—2 treatments down and 4 to go—a third of the way through this part of the treatment!

Of course the amount of saline administered means that according to the nurse "she will pee like a racehorse for a while" which I must admit conjures up pictures of my wife going to the loo standing astride in the field at the back of our house! Or maybe I misunderstood her?

Anyway that's the update for today, and please don't take this the wrong way, but I really hope the blog will be quiet for a few days now and that we have less drama with the side effects than last time. But then again—remember our mantra—expect the unexpected!

10

Telling the Children

So five days into the second round of chemo and so far so good. Miranda is feeling OK, a little nauseous from time to time but generally not too bad. Of course it is over the next few days that she may start to really feel the effects of the chemo so I don't want to tempt fate. "Expect the unexpected" constantly rings in my ears! We are hoping that this time however, she will avoid going neutropenic as 24 hours after her last chemo she had an injection of a very clever drug that will lay dormant inside her and only kick in when her white blood count plummets. Amazing!

I thought therefore it was an opportunity to talk about a key part of our "journey" so far.

We have two wonderful girls and I think one of the toughest things about this disease has been getting our heads around how we tell them of the challenge facing their Mum and support them through the months ahead. At just 5 and 2 years old they are so, so young to have to face this and Rose, our eldest, has just completed her first term at school. She's loved it and we have seen her confidence and social skills blossom so much over the past three months. We both want so much to ensure that this illness doesn't impact upon her development at school.

So when Miranda was diagnosed we both quickly focussed on how we would tell them. And the first thing we agreed is that there isn't really a right or wrong way and, to a certain extent, you have to go with a "gut feel" on what feels right. So this is how we told our children but please remember this is our story and we would hate to give the impression that we think this is how everyone faced with this most challenging of tasks should do it. And of course it is far too early to determine whether what we have done is right or has worked for our two.

Firstly we told the school—we felt that they would be in a great position to notice any changes in Rose's behaviour or if she seemed to be different or quieter and that would be helpful for them to know the possible cause and to alert us to the change in her behaviour.

With Miranda being diagnosed just before Christmas we had to decide whether to tell them before or after the festivities. In the end we felt that we would tell them before, given that we weren't certain how we, or our parents, would deal with Christmas given the shock of the news. We didn't want the children picking up on any tension or upset and not knowing why it was there.

We also felt that we didn't want to make a big production of the news. Sitting them down specially to tell them with both of us present we felt might make them nervous as we've never done that type of "family summit" before. Miranda also felt that she wanted to be the one to tell them and so we agreed that the news would be introduced when the three of them sat down to have their tea.

There were a few things that we both felt were important—firstly we had to be completely honest in what we told them and in any answers we gave to questions they may have. You can't sugar coat "Mummy's got cancer." But more importantly if we make promises to them that we don't know whether will come true or not then we felt we risked losing their trust and confidence in us.

So basically Miranda reminded them about the recent visits she had to the hospital and that the Doctors were trying to find out why she has some lumps in her neck, under her arm and in her boob and that they had found something growing inside her that shouldn't be there. She explained that she would need to have some medicine and that although initially the lump wouldn't make Mummy poorly the medicine would, but that if she didn't have the medicine then she would eventually get very poorly indeed. And that the Doctors were confident that by having the medicine the lump would go and Mummy would eventually be better.

Miranda told them about some of the side effects too. Rose has had experience of cancer in that one of her ballet teachers had recently has breast cancer and so Miranda was able to explain that Mummy would lose her hair like Helen.

And when Miranda had finished explaining all this Rose said "OK Mummy—could you pass me that decoration off the Christmas tree—I want to have a look at it!!" Aren't children just the best!

So the news was out and since then we have tried to ensure we find a balance between keeping them involved and aware of what is happening but also ensuring that the cancer doesn't take over our lives. We need to ensure they understand the "new normal" of how our life is and appreciate some of the benefits that this new normal brings. Like the fact that Grandma will be staying more regularly and that Daddy will be home for more bathtimes and bedtime stories. I'd like to think they are still young enough to see that last one as a good thing!

We've used some of the excellent resources provided by the Macmillan Trust to guide us. Apparently a common reaction in children the age of our two is to feel that the illness is "their fault" or to get angry at the person who is ill for not giving them the same attention as normal. So we have tried to give them lots of reassurance.

Our plan is to keep them involved and we expected to take Rose on one of the chemo days so that she can see for herself what having the medicine involves for her Mum. However after the reaction Miranda had at the last session we might have to take a raincheck on this idea for a while.

Generally they seem to have taken things in their stride and the only time either of them have shown any signs of struggling with the situation is when Miranda has suddenly disappeared into hospital overnight but I think that is to be expected. Millie is too young to really have any conversation with on this subject but I make sure that Rose and I just catch up on how we are doing and what she is thinking. I've asked her about her Mum's wig—"Mummy looks beautiful Daddy"—and of course she is absolutely right. We pray together for her Mum some nights too. The only time she has complained is when she had to go back to school after the holidays while Miranda was in hospital. "It's just not fair Daddy all the other children have their Mummys if they need them but me and Millie don't" Cue for a few tears . . . . I think Rose might have cried at that point too but I can't really remember!

So that is the story with the children so far. It's difficult and probably too early to tell how we are doing and that is quite a scary situation to be in. I am convinced that they will respond to our determination to remain upbeat and positive throughout but who knows . . . .

As I've mentioned before we're on a journey and we've never been on this path before—I so don't want us to lose our way.

11

There's No One Quite Like Grandma

As some of you will know, up until now we have been able to maintain our "normal life" over the two weeks of the chemo programme when Miranda is most likely to feel at her worst, thanks to my mother-in-law, Barbara who flies in (not on her broomstick—who said that?!) from her home near Stratford-upon-Avon to stay with us. She has been a wonderful help and so, so supportive of the four of us.

I have to admit that I struck gold in the mother-in-law stakes; she is a great cook, being a former teacher is wonderful with our children (who, in return, clearly love their Grandma) and, best of all, get this—she loves football, is a huge cricket fan and even used to be a scorer for the village side in her younger days! I mean who could ask for more—although it is a bit of a shame that she's a Lincoln City fan who also has a slight preference for Coventry City too (being her local side) but I'm prepared to overlook this minor faux pas. And, given the current furore, let me reassure you that she absolutely knows the offside law and all its nuances. As the much maligned, now former Sky Sports commentator, Andy Gray might say, "take a bow son"—or maybe in this new world of complete political correctness it should be "take a curtsy Grandma"!!

Anyway disaster has struck, Grandma's not very well. She's had a really nasty cold and just couldn't make it down. Given that this week should be Miranda's toughest we've been a little nervous as to how we might cope. However thanks to the wonder of the extra injection Miranda had, and the power of prayer, she has had a remarkably good week. The challenges of the last round of chemo with the swollen mouth, horrible rash and regular temperatures have not materialised and we are almost through the week flying solo without the safety net of Grandma. It means that Grandma can have a full two weeks off before we need her back again. But we have all missed her.

In the interests of balance I would also like to point out that I do have a great father-in-law too, not least because he allows us to have Barbara on loan for such long periods!

Clearly it's still been a hard week for Miranda but she has been much more ready to listen to her body and take it easy when necessary. She is even getting better at asking for help—asking friends to take Rose to school when she hasn't felt up to it or, as was the case this morning, just simply overslept!! This time around the side effects seem to have materialised as a horrible taste in her mouth, a strange tongue sensation, hands feeling burnt and the occasional feeling that breathing is more of an effort. This horrible taste in her mouth has meant that it has been impossible to drink wine (disaster!), beetroot soup (no great loss!), but amazingly chocolate and cake have still gone down remarkably easily. She felt really poorly on Tuesday evening (I think this might be that she was just missing me as I'd headed down to the Emirates to see the valiant Tractor Boys of Ipswich take on Arsenal in the Carling Cup Semi-Final!) but still decided to go to our regular weekly get together with some of our friends from the Forge on the basis that one of them was a GP so she was in the perfect place if things really took a turn for the worse.

Obviously I have got involved with more of the parenting tasks at the weekend and last Saturday morning took Rose to her ballet class leaving Miranda and Millie cuddling in bed. Rose loves ballet but I have to say I am a bit of a novice at such matters as this was her first Saturday class having previously gone on a Thursday after school when I was at work. Having arrived early at the venue we then had a major drama of putting on her ballet shoes—who'd thought something that appears so simple could be so complicated—I swallowed all pride in the end and asked a nearby Mum to "coach" me in the intricacies and Rose was ready. Or not actually—she now decided she needed the toilet just as the class was about to start. After much rushing around I shepherded her into the class just as the teacher was about to begin the first moves. With a sigh of relief I moved to the parents area only to realise to my horror that I had inadvertently tucked her cardigan into the top of her skirt. I then suffered an agonising 10 minutes of trying to attract Rose's attention but failing before the ballet teacher finally noticed and made the necessary adjustments. Then 30 minutes into the 45 minute class Rose uncharacteristically burst into tears for no apparent reason. The ballet teacher, Sandra, comforted her and then suggested, rather helpfully, that perhaps it would be a good idea if Daddy joined in! Oh deep, deep joy! Can I just say that for someone who probably carries a few pounds more than he should I felt I was remarkably light on my feet and furthermore, mastered the very intricate steps of the routine with unexpected ease. This class is so advanced for 5 year olds you know! Sandra—I know you read this blog—do feel free to leave a compliment—sorry I mean comment—on my ballet skills. I have to say though that I could, of course, tell that you were secretly quite impressed!

Meanwhile Miranda has felt up to have her bird watching friend around to put up nets and "ring" the birds in our garden as part of a large Suffolk Wildlife project.

By now you can tell that we both believe in living life on the edge can't you?!

So this weekend we head into week three of round two of chemo and it should be a better week for Miranda as the side effects of the chemo diminish. We've got a good weekend lined up with Philip, one of my best friends, coming up from London to stay with us. Now, that's got me thinking . . . I wonder what he's like at ballet? Over to you Sandra!

12

Islington & the IRA: Influences on My Childhood

So another week has flown by and I'm sat in front of a roaring fire with a glass of wine (makes the words flow that much easier I find!) and realising it's high time to update the blog. It's been a pretty uneventful week to be honest—which is great! It's Miranda's final week of this chemo cycle so she should be at her strongest and that's pretty much how it has been, save for a nasty 48 hour virus that seems to have hit both of us. It left us feeling pretty rough for a while and I even had to have a day off work which is a rare occurrence indeed. The weekend brings a family wedding which, given the circumstances, the West Country location and the consequent long journey I'm attending without the three girls. I am not alone for the weekend though, I am travelling down with my Mum.

Miranda is certainly getting used to her wig although there was a memorable moment this week when as they rushed out the door to make it to school Rose suddenly said "Mummy—what about your hair!" Never mind having a bad hair day—she nearly had a no hair day!

Both children are still coping remarkably well although, without a doubt, we are starting to see some inevitable impact on Rose who clearly now worries more about being ill herself and gets upset at the thought of having a headache and the like. We have to be discerning to work out whether she really is genuinely ill or just worried about being ill. When the virus got me on Monday I felt pretty awful as I put Rose to bed so I let her know that I might not go to work the next day. "Daddy you're not going to be poorly like Mummy are you?" she asked with a look of fear in her eyes that made my blood run cold. I reassured her that I would be just fine very soon and then we hugged goodnight, holding each other far tighter and for far longer than we usually do.

I've got to be honest the impact this illness will have on our children is still something that bothers me as much as anything and it is this thought that makes me the most angry at times. I'm so cross that they have to experience this and I do worry about the permanent impact that it will have on their development. It's led me, more than once, to think about my own childhood and the experiences that shaped and influenced me . . . .

For all my childhood, and about thirty years in total, my Dad owned a Sub-Post Office on Goswell Road in Islington, pretty much halfway between the Angel and the Barbican for those of you who know London. It was the days before the complete traffic mayhem and congestion charging that now exists in our capital city. So the evening routine was that Mum and I would eat around 6:30pm and Dad would arrive home somewhere between 6:45pm and 7pm and have his dinner slightly behind us and we'd sit and talk for a bit, maybe watch some telly and then it was my bedtime. Except one night just before Christmas in 1975 Dad didn't turn up. I was ten but I can remember the events as they unfurled as though it was just a week or so ago. By 7:30pm Mum and I were really concerned. No mobile phones in those days so I just spent the whole time looking out our front window at the stream of traffic hoping against hope that one of the approaching car headlights would start indicating and turn into our drive. As I write this I can still remember the tight feeling in the pit of my stomach that I had that night. Around 8pm the phone rang and it was the police asking if Dad could go to the shop as they had reports of a break in. Mum explained that he hadn't turned up and was effectively missing. She rang a member of his staff who lived in Turnpike House, a high rise block of flats opposite Dad's shop, and they went to check the shop and the whereabouts of Dad's car with the police. The shop was unlocked and empty and Dad's car was in the underground car park where he had left it that morning. A full scale police operation started to find Dad and understand why the shop was as it was. I remember at this point my Mum just collapsing in floods of tears and I can remember going through the thought process that I mustn't cry too or that would make my Mum worse.

The mid 70's was when the IRA were at their most active in London with bombing campaigns and it transpired that an active IRA cell needing to fund their campaign had put Dad's shop under surveillance. They learnt his routine at the 5:30pm closing time. They parked their van next to his car in the underground car park and when he got to his car that night they jumped him, bundled him into the back of the van, bound, gagged and beat him up. Three guys stayed with him while a couple of others went back to the shop, opened it up and went in with the intention of robbing the post office. The lock on the door between the shop and the post office was a bit sticky and in their haste and panic they couldn't get it open and assumed Dad had told them the wrong key for the lock. So they went back to the van and beat him up some more, they threatened to put him in a sack and throw him in the Thames. Dad assured them it was the right key and implored them to let him go across and help them open up. He'd told them the right key but bravely (or stupidly) told them the wrong combination to the safe. They didn't trust him so they went back to the shop and tried again. They failed and back they went for more beating and threats—this process carried on for four more attempts and lasted about two hours. Eventually a passer-by who knew Dad challenged them as they were at the shop entrance and they were unnerved and gave up. They drove Dad away in the van and left him tied up in the back of it. Badly beaten, minus numerous teeth and bound so tightly that the bruises on his arms stayed visible for weeks he eventually managed to kick his way out of the van and raise the alarm. It was five hours after his ordeal started and at 10pm we got the call to say Dad was safe. My Mum stopped crying and I remember that the relief was overwhelming and knowing that all was OK I was released and able to cry. So I did—like I've never cried before or since. And when my Dad got home just after midnight I hugged him far tighter and for far longer than normal—just like I hugged Rose on Monday in fact.

I tell you that powerful story as I realise that the impact it had on me was immense. I worried a lot more about my Dad, worried about being attacked, worried about being alone in dark and, up until his passing three years ago, I couldn't tolerate anyone saying anything bad about him. I grew up with less confidence and was far more nervous as a teenager than I think I would have been if I hadn't gone through this experience. But I also saw my Dad's immense bravery, he was back at work the next day, he still parked his car in the underground car park for months until the council found him a street parking space. And he never displayed any anger he just simply taught me that what counts is not how many times you get knocked down in life but how many times you get up. He lived out a brave, humble response to this terrible experience with little animosity towards his attackers. His response has shaped and influenced who I am too.

Now I know that my Mum and Dad must have hated the fact I had to go through that night, must have worried about the impact it would have on me and would have given anything to have shielded me from it. Just as Miranda and I hate the fact that Rose and Millie have to go through this illness, worry about the impact it will have on them and would give anything to shield them from it. But we can't—it's real life. Terrorists, muggers and beatings are real life, nasty lumps growing under your skin are real life, drugs that can make you better but also make you feel really sick and all your hair fall out are real life.

These life lessons have come early for our two just as it did for me on that December night in 1975. But as I was reminded in a recent talk at the Forge, our ultimate responsibility as parents is not to create a perfect, wonderful happy childhood for our children but to prepare them for adult life—to get them as strong, disciplined and wise as we can, to face all the many challenges that adult life will throw at them. So this experience that we are all going through is an opportunity for us to prepare Rose and Millie, to demonstrate how we tackle adversity and we need to gracefully accept that it will have a negative impact on them too but that is real life. And when it gets a bit tough, well, we will just have to hug them a bit tighter and for a bit longer than we normally do—and guess what, that's actually a really wonderful thing to do!

13

Live in the Chemo Club Lounge

So today I'm writing this live in the "Chemo Club Lounge" whilst Miranda has her third dose of chemotherapy. In fact today, as she had such a bad reaction last time, we are just off the Club Lounge and in the VIP suite—so that she can get better attention and also, largely, I expect, so that we don't freak out the others in the lounge if she has another bad reaction!

Before Miranda got this disease I had no real concept of what receiving chemotherapy was like and so I thought I would while away the time today by telling you a little bit about what it is like on the inside. I've named the chemotherapy day unit at Ipswich Hospital as the "chemo club lounge" as it really does have the feel of a club. We all sit around on comfortable chairs the only thing distinguishing between relatives and patients being the location of the drip stand, the pillow on your lap and a canula in your arm! We are also provided with magazines, a coffee machine (although I much prefer the walk down to Costa Coffee at the other end of the hospital!) and an army of nurses to look after us! Without doubt the nature of why we are all here adds a certain camaraderie amongst the patients and an unspoken look of mutual support and understanding of what each other is going through.

I never appreciated that chemotherapy was so complex and that everybody has a different recipe with a huge range of different drugs used. This means that people come and go at different times although it is fair to say that given Miranda's challenges with the chemo we are usually amongst the first to arrive and have always been the last to leave!

Just off from the "club lounge" is an area in a corridor where presumably those who are having slightly less potent drugs are all sat being treated. Given that this is our third visit I have never seen less than 6 people in the corridor area and never less than 5 people in the lounge at any one time—you start to realise the scale of impact of this disease. There is a whiteboard that the nurses use in the corridor and this morning I counted 32 people in for some form of chemotherapy today and that's just in the day ward on one day. Wow!

Between the corridor treatment area and the lounge is a room where they actually prepare and mix the chemicals. I am fascinated by this room to be honest. There are a team of pharmacists on the go all the time we've been here and the potency of the chemo drugs demands that they put their hands through two tubes and mix them behind a glass screen in an enclosed environment. Each patient literally does have their own chemo recipe and clearly these are made to order on the day. Somehow I just never thought that the chemo drugs would be so individual and actually made up on site.

And I need to also mention the nurses—we've mainly been looked after by Helen, Charlotte and Claire and they are all really wonderful, fitting the stereotype of the hard working, caring nurse with a genuine desire to care for their patients. Every nurse seems to work so hard and their help and support when Miranda had her reaction last time was first class. Fortunately, from my perspective, they are also happy to humour me with some banter which is a core part of my coping strategy! In one of those strange quirks of fate it transpires that Charlotte, who is getting married in April, has recently won a competition for a free wedding at Ufford Park which is where we operate the spa and health club. As part of her prize she gets a spa day too and I'm so going to make sure that our team look after her!

We're now back in the main lounge as Miranda's not had any reaction to the drugs so far and sadly another poor lady has. She needs to be moved into the "VIP" cubicle where we were as it has a bed that she can recover on. It's not the most pleasant experience having chemo at the best of times but when it goes wrong it really is quite horrible.

So I look around the lounge and what hits me, just as it did the first couple of times we came in, is that I can be confident that at least half the people in the room receiving treatment are younger than me and a couple are younger than Miranda. The diversity of the people here is incredible, all brought together in one room by one horrible disease. Last time we were here we got talking to a lady who is in her sixties—she was so friendly and pleasant—but was really amazed that we lived in Suffolk and didn't own a boat! Her upbringing and experience of Suffolk was just so different to our own. She was on her 4th chemo cycle. When she went home her chair was taken by a young Portuguese lady who had three children and a husband who also acted as interpreter for her as she didn't speak a word of English. They had come over here in search of work and he struggled to get time off to accompany her and they were panicking about getting home in time to get their children from school. It was only her second visit and her fear was palpable.

It has just brought home to me that cancer is no respecter of age, wealth, education, lifestyle or upbringing. One day it just happens, randomly, and suddenly you find yourself with a paid up subscription to the chemo club lounge and membership with a group of people that, but for this disease, you would never have encountered.

Well I'm pleased to report that we are now ready to leave. The third chemo has been administered and Miranda is fine and we are not, for once, the last to head out of the lounge. In fact we will have time to pop into Ipswich and I'm so pleased and relieved at how well behaved my wife has been today that I might have to treat her to something from "White Stuff", her favourite clothing store. The fact that I might check out the men's section too and that the shop is directly opposite Starbucks is one of those happy coincidences!

We now just have to hope that the next three weeks are as plain sailing as the last three have been. Before I sign off I want to leave you with one parting thought. Every time I walk down the stairs at our house there is a phrase carved into a block of wood on the shelves to my left that reads:

> *"Life is not measured by the number of breaths we take, but by the moments that take our breath away"*

With all what has happened over the past couple of months and after spending some time in the "Chemo Club Lounge" I'm so determined that I will engineer some "moments to take my breath away" for me, and for Miranda and the girls, as often as possible.

I really hope that reading this blog encourages you to do the same.

14

Hold on Fast

So what are you doing Tuesday? It's Miranda's birthday—it would be rude and wrong of me to tell you how old she will be and I can think of oooh, let me think, well at least 37 reasons why I shouldn't?! I'm not sure she will be up for much of a celebration to be honest as she feels pretty rubbish at the moment. This is only to be expected given the stage of the chemo cycle she is at but the horrible mouth, strange taste, nausea and general sense of feeling wiped out is back with a vengeance right now. As ever, of course, she is putting on her brave face and just getting on with life as normal. Quite amazing really.

Anyway, as I have mentioned before we are part of the Forge Community Church which meets in Debenham, Suffolk. I just wanted to let all of you know that this Tuesday The Forge is holding a special day of prayer for healing for Miranda, two other people from the Church who also have cancer and another young guy who has a rare condition that affects his ability to cope with heat. It is yet another example of how incredibly supportive The Forge has been to us through this difficult time.

As well as praying, a number of people will also be fasting—going without food for 24 hours. This will probably seem to be a rather unusual thing to do but there are clear biblical and spiritual reasons for so doing. In this instance the purpose of fasting is to show God that we are serious about what we are asking for and that we don't want to take "no" for an answer. Clearly fasting is only appropriate in certain situations and for certain people. Some people with certain medical conditions or who are pregnant definitely shouldn't fast.

But Miranda and I wanted to just use this blog to thank those of you from the Forge for supporting us in this way and to give those of you who are not part of the Forge but would like to take part in the day of prayer and fasting the chance to do so.

We recognise of course that many of you will not feel inclined to take part and we fully understand and appreciate that and wouldn't want you to feel in anyway obliged to. Support for us has manifested itself in so many ways—through practical ways of cooking us meals, helping with the children or jobs around the house but also through many ways of encouragement in cards, letters, texts, emails, comments on this blog, phone calls and conversations. We value all of them and consider ourselves very blessed to have had so much support and Tuesday is yet one more way of that support being expressed.

Tomorrow is our wedding anniversary so I think that is definitely worthy of a blog don't you? See you here tomorrow then!

15

Love Actually

Given that I actually got the name for this blog from a scene in one of his films, I'm sure that Richard Curtis won't mind me borrowing the title of one of his other films for this post. But you see the past week has all been about love. Last weekend I went to the wedding of my cousin Ben to Lucy and today is my own wedding anniversary!

So today kicks off a three day celebration festival in our household, wedding anniversary today, Valentine's Day tomorrow and then my wife's birthday the day after! The great thing about this is that there really is no chance of forgetting these events, a stereotypical male faux pas, sandwiching Valentine's Day as they do. The downside is finding a different, meaningful and innovative way to write "I love you" in a card on the third consecutive day and, of course, making sure I give the appropriate card on the right day. I still dread getting the day of Miranda's birthday and our anniversary the wrong way around!

But let's go back to last week's wedding. I come from a really small family. Although I was fortunate to grow up with both my parents happily married to each other, I'm an only child and had one Aunt, one Uncle, one cousin and, for all bar my first five years, one Grandparent. So although Bev, my cousin, grew up 200 miles away from me (I was in London and Bev in Devon) we spent our annual holiday at her house in Devon and they visited us every Christmas and we've grown up together. We've both gone through some tough times as adults, Bev's lost both her parents and I've lost my Dad and over the last few years we've grown closer and I admire so much what Bev has achieved in her life despite some significant challenges. Being an only child I've no concept of what it's like to have a sister but Bev's the closest I've got, save for Miranda's wonderful sister Lou obviously, and for a cousin she makes a fantastic sister if you know what I mean! So it was great to see her last weekend at her son Ben's wedding.

The fact that Bev was barely in her 20's when she had her first child, and that I was just into my 40's when Rose was born, means that our children are a generation apart. Bev's eldest, Chloe, is 27, whilst Ben, who got married, is 24, and Vicky is 19. I suppose I tend to think of the three of them as more like nieces and nephews (rather than the second cousins that they actually are) and they are all great people. Suffice to say if Rose and Millie turn out to be the adults that Chloe and Vicky are, I will consider myself to be very blessed and very proud.

The wedding itself was just the most spectacular I've ever been to. The whole event was staged at a beautiful country house—think Downton Abbey meets Hogwarts—just a stones throw from the West Country coast in a village near Minehead. The day started with the ceremony itself in a beautiful Orangery set in manicured gardens, followed by a champagne and canapé reception with an excellent wedding singer to entertain. The wedding breakfast that followed was lovely, the speeches were short (phew!), the favours and table decorations like I've never seen before. And of all of this was followed with a professional firework display (incredible but I dread to think what it cost!), a hog roast and evening entertainment. What a day!

Now given that, prior to meeting Miranda, my track record in the marriage stakes was nothing short of abysmal I'm not in a position to offer Ben and Lucy any advice about how to make their marriage work but this much I do know. What I will remember most of all about their special day, long after the memory of the spectacular venue, the fireworks, five tier cake and seven bridesmaids has faded, took place in the ceremony itself. Ben and Lucy decided to have their own vows which they had written, learnt and declared to each other in front of all of us. Those vows were incredibly personal and spoken with an obvious love in their eyes, a sense of joy in their hearts and perhaps, most importantly of all, a real conviction in their voices.

Very, very special.

I really hope they keep a copy of those vows somewhere safe so that when the inevitable challenging times that all couples face at some point occurs, they can get those vows back out and remind themselves of what they promised and committed to each other. It will stand them in such good stead.

Inevitably Ben and Lucy's vows reminded me of those I made to Miranda, exactly six years ago today. It's such a shame that I'm getting so much practice at putting the "in sickness" bit into action right now but that is just how it is. I made those vows, I meant them then, I mean them now and no matter how tough it gets I am so determined to fulfil those vows over the months and years ahead.

Amongst the many traditions of the wedding day is the newlyweds first dance and as I watched Ben and Lucy take to the floor for theirs, I'll admit to a bit of a lump in the throat. Probably mainly because the build up to a floor full of people brought home to me that I was on my own as Miranda wasn't up to making the long trip and had stayed at home with our girls. It was also I suspect because I had a flashback to being in my early 20's and rather awkwardly holding this beautiful baby boy and it seemed incongruous that this tiny baby was now taking to the dance floor with his bride. I also therefore did the inevitable projecting forward to a possible day in the future when one of my girls may be making that same dance and well—oh boy—can't imagine how I will deal with that! And finally it was because it reminded me of a story from a book I've just started by one of my favourite authors, John Ortberg, called "The Me I Want To Be." By the way if you ever get the chance to read his book "When the Game is Over It All Goes Back in the Box" you should do; it is so challenging and thought provoking. But right now I want to share this story from the book with you. Ortberg writes:

> "My niece Courtney got married not long ago, and at the wedding reception they had a dance for married couples in which they would eliminate couples from the dance floor based on the length of their marriage. At the beginning we were all on the floor. Courtney and Patrick were the first to leave, then all the couples married less than one year left, then those married less than five years, and so on. Nancy and I made it to the twenty-five-year cut, and by that time the crowd had thinned out considerably.
>
> Finally, there was only one couple left on the dance floor, and they had been married fifty-three years. Everybody watched them—a tall, courtly, silver-haired man who stood a foot taller than his wife—but they watched only each other. They danced with joy, not in the skill of their dancing, but in the love they radiated for each other. What

a contrast between the newlyweds, fresh in the health and beauty of their marriage, and the beauty of another kind of love that shone from the last couple on the floor! Perhaps part of why we appreciate such beauty is that it speaks to us of an inner flourishing not visible to the eye.

When the dancing ended, the master of ceremonies turned to Courtney and Patrick and said to them, "Take a good look at that couple on that dance floor. Your task now is to live and love together in such a way that fifty-three years from now that's you. That dance is your dance. Now it begins."

So Miranda and I have been dancing that dance for six years and let me tell you that every step has been as wonderful and magical as I hoped and thought it would be. Obviously there have been times when I've been a bit clumsy and out of step—those of you who have seen me on the dance floor will not be at all surprised at this I know—but each time that's happened Miranda has gently brought back into line. So I will continue this dance with my beautiful bride remembering that no matter what difficult steps we have to face we will dance our way through them with sheer determination and smiles on our faces. I can assure you that we will be on the dance floor for a very long time yet.

Happy Anniversary Sweetheart—just can't find the words to tell you how much I love you! Not today, nor tomorrow (Valentine's Day) nor the day after (your birthday) either! But I think you know I do, don't you!

16

Climb Every Mountain

So let's start this week's post with the some really good news. As she is approaching the halfway stage of this section of the chemo treatment, Miranda has been back to the hospital this week for some scans and a mammogram to assess how effective treatment has been so far. The immediate feedback is that there is a significant reduction in the size of the tumour and that the lymph nodes in her neck are back to normal size. This is just wonderful news and was obviously what we had hoped for. The power of prayer and medicine combined!

It is good too that Miranda has suffered far less dramatically from the side effects of the chemo this time around than she did after the first dose. That's not to say that she hasn't felt pretty ropey on some days and that she hasn't experienced any side effects. We were warned about the potency of the chemo drug and that it can cause problems with the veins into which it is injected. This week the vein in her left hand, which has received two of the doses so far, is visibly burnt by the chemicals and she has a nasty sore, red vein all the way up to the crease of her elbow. Nasty and more proof were any needed, that these drugs are powerful!

We also had some excitement on her birthday when her heart, without warning and for no apparent reason, suddenly starting beating fast and raced up to approximately 200 beats per minute. An emergency trip to the doctor ensued and the incident was put down to a supraventricular tachycardia (!) which in layman's terms means the electrical currents in the heart getting out of synch. The net result is that Miranda was left feeling very tired from the experience and she has to have her heart rate monitored for 24hours this week. Bizarrely this may just be some random event and not linked to the chemo at all. I know she gets excited on her birthday but this was a bit extreme to be honest!

Of course Miranda has, as ever, dealt with this with her usual humour, determination and bravery. Indeed, to be honest, those who she encounters in everyday life could be forgiven for not realising exactly what she is going through. For me, however, this week has been a bit of a slog. And I'm not sure quite why. It could be the fact that we've not really been able to celebrate our anniversary and Miranda's birthday, it could be because it's been a long, tough week at work or it could be because we're almost at the milestone of halfway in the first stage of treatment and there's the realisation that we still have so much ahead of us. Anyway, whatever the cause, my "positivity tanks" have been running on close to empty.

For some reason this lack of energy has made me cast my mind back to last summer when I undertook the 3 Peaks Challenge—walking the 3 highest peaks in Britain (Ben Nevis, Scar Fell and Snowdon) in 24 hours. Given that I'd never even climbed one mountain before in my life this could be viewed as brave, or stupid, or both perhaps. But I did it—and it was just a brilliant thing to do. I learnt so much on that walk about myself and about life and I need to draw on those lessons right now I think.

Looking back the two most memorable moments were getting to the top of Ben Nevis and the awful weather as I laboured up Snowdon. As you may know Ben Nevis is the highest mountain and so getting to the top brought a real sense of achievement. Despite the fact that we did the climb in June the top of the mountain was still covered in snow but the weather was glorious and the view completely clear at the summit. As I looked around the mountain range it was simply a stunning view—a "creation appreciation" moment the like of which I have never experienced before. I took some photos but they just don't do justice to the sheer beauty of the evening sun bouncing off the incredible white topped mountains that we looked down on. Breathtaking doesn't really adequately convey the scene that unfurled in front of me.

But the other memorable moment on that walk was when I got halfway up Snowdon. The weather couldn't have been more different to that on Ben Nevis. Driving wind and throwing it down with rain. I was 21 hours into the adventure, had climbed two mountains already and had grabbed just two hours sleep in the car between mountains so it's fair to say I wasn't at my most sprightly. The rain was washing the dried on sweat that covered my face into my eyes making it difficult to see. I was scrabbling over rocks and began to doubt that I could make it to the top. I'd already learnt from the earlier climbs that what appeared to be the top of the mountain was probably not and behind the summit in view would be further higher summits to climb to get to the mountain top. So I stopped, grabbed a Mars bar and banana from my rucksack (great instant energy food by the way) and gave myself a bit of a talking to before continuing on and making it to the top within the 24 hour deadline. It was a powerful lesson about how important it is to just keep going when the toughest thing to do is actually to just keep going.

I also think the experience on those mountains and with that journey will stand me in good stead for this journey with Miranda's battle with cancer. You see I know this too is going to be a tough journey. I also know that the "summit" we see ahead is probably not the last summit we have to reach but that there are many rewards to enjoy from the journey too. We've received so much love and practical help from friends, our children have a much closer relationship with their Grandma than would otherwise have been possible and we have drawn closer together as a family.

You see what I've also learnt is this. Did I want to stand, walk, and at times, crawl up a mountain in the pounding rain? No! Was that part of the actual experience one I would describe as pleasant? Obviously not! But do I, looking back, regret making that climb and going through that experience? Of course not. I'm so glad I did that walk, met that challenge and experienced all the things I did including that tough climb on Snowdon. I look back on it with a sense of pride, achievement and, without doubt, it was a memorable journey. Maybe one day, sometime ahead of now, when we've reached the final summit of this current journey we're on, we will all look back on the experience, on our time living with cancer and feel exactly the same way.

So please excuse me but before I continue the journey I need to head off and get myself a Mars bar and a banana.

17

Visiting Time

So half term has brought the usual stream of visitors to the house—we both love entertaining! We had a great time last weekend with our friend Naomi coming to stay. Naomi and husband Julian have two daughters similar in age to ours and we got to know them through the ante-natal course we both attended when Rose was born. We had just the best time with Naomi and both our girls, especially Rose, love being around her and Miranda too is always in a much better frame of mind for spending time with her. Of all our friends Naomi also has the best ever claim to fame . . . . but I promised I wouldn't put details in the blog or I would be Busted—ooh that's a clue actually! You will have to let me know if you want the full story! It's a good one I promise.

With Naomi's departure came the arrival of Miranda's sister Lou and our nieces, Chloe and Sophie. They are simply the best nieces anyone could wish for and together with their Mum, Lou, are just three more reasons why it is so great to be married to Miranda! In fact their visit is worthy of a blog post on its own so I'll tell you all about that next time as they are still staying with us.

Miranda has had her 24 hour heart rate assessment. Electrodes were placed on her heart and a monitor recorded every beat whilst attached to her belt. She had to record any activity she took and when she ate and we will wait to see what the results show and whether they in anyway indicate why she suffered last week's episode. I still can't believe that I managed to get through the whole time she was wearing it without once hiding behind a door and jumping out at the last moment shouting "boo" at the top of my voice just to see the effect it had. But somehow I did—hope you are impressed with me?!

This is a week when Miranda feels at her best so we are making the most of it and I'm having the day off tomorrow to go to see "Shaun the Sheep" in Norwich—I think the girls are a bit more excited than me but it's a close run thing! Friday night we are off out for a belated birthday and anniversary celebration—can't wait! And Saturday night we are off to friends for one of those murder mystery dinner party nights. Miranda is organising the costumes and I wait with interest to see who I am playing! Our social calendar has never seemed so hectic!

And then Monday it's back to the hospital for round 4 of the chemo treatment and off we go again. I'm afraid there will be no stories from me in the chemo club lounge this time as I'm skiving off—I'm at a Spa Conference in London with some meetings that were difficult to get out of. Is that really bad of me? Yes? Thought you'd say that. Expect another blog update from me next week when my tail will probably still be firmly between my legs! And assuming of course that the murder mystery evening doesn't get too out of hand!

18

Reasons to be Cheerful

I guarantee those of you of the same vintage as me will have read the title of this post and then in your head said "one—two—three" in your best Ian Dury and the Blockheads impression! The rest of you will, of course, have no idea what I'm talking about.

Anyway on with the post. I've a friend who works with me—she does an amazing job looking after our IT systems and produces reports daily on the performance of our spas. She also has a great blog which I always try to keep up to date with. One of the features of Clare's blog is that every Friday she posts at least three reasons to be cheerful. It's a kind of upbeat, good news way to end the week and I think it is a really clever idea to ensure we all look for the many positives that are always around us but sometimes just need teasing out a little bit more some weeks than others! So on the basis that imitation is the best form of flattery I've stolen Clare's idea and here are my reasons to be cheerful this weekend—ready—one—two—three:

One: The best reason to be cheerful is that my sister-in-law Lou and her two daughters Chloe and Sophie came to stay with us for three days this week. Although I had to work and didn't get that much time with them, all three are really wonderful and it was just great to catch up. We don't see as much of them as we'd like as they live in Oxford, we seem to always have so much on whilst Lou, and husband Ju, both work shifts meaning that it is a logistical challenge to find space in all four diaries. So when we do see them it makes it that much more special. Our two daughters get on really well with their cousins, Chloe and Sophie. There is only five weeks between Rose and Sophie in age and this time around they really seemed to love playing together. I always know when our two girls have had fun with visitors to the house as the conversation about them carries on after the guests have left and, still this morning, both Rose and Millie were talking about their cousins. It is so good that they get on so well. For Chloe and Sophie I think it was good for them to see Auntie Minnie (their name for Miranda). They know she's not well and so it was a chance for them to understand that a bit better and to see at first hand that she is doing just fine and carrying on as normal. They actually unintentionally saw her without her wig and although it unnerved them a tiny bit, the incident enabled them to ask a few more questions and for Lou to give them some reassurance. All in all it was a great time.

It goes without saying that Miranda valued so much seeing her sister too but it was also good for me to catch up with Lou over dinner most evenings. We now share a common bond of having to be bystanders whilst we watch someone we both love very much go through this horrible battle with cancer. Miranda had a few hours at music practice one night so Lou and I had the chance to talk about how we are coping. Miranda's illness will inevitably draw us even closer together and so this week it was so good that we got some time to eat, talk a bit, drink some wine, laugh a lot and cry a little. We probably needed to do all those things together.

I really love my nieces and my sister-in-law very much. And what I love most of all is that I have the type of relationship with Lou where we can be totally honest and real with each other. She has been so supportive to both me and Miranda, often just through the things she says, and over the last few days Lou has gently taught me how I can improve the way I'm handling this situation. I need that and I love her all the more for the way she is "journeying" with us. It has been a very good week indeed.

Two: The second reason to be cheerful is that Miranda and I managed to get a night out together, just the two of us, on Friday night. Time out as a couple is so precious these days and so difficult to schedule in. Friday night enabled us to talk on a level that we can't when the children are around or when we are tired on a week night. I know that we need time like that to keep our marriage on track and Friday night was also special as it served as a delayed birthday, anniversary and valentine celebration all rolled into one.

We went to the Galley in Woodbridge which, if I was forced to choose one, I would probably have as my favourite all time restaurant. There's a Galley in Ipswich too and we used to be regulars at both locations prior to the arrival of the children and the curtailing of our nights out! I always get inspired when I go there, not just by the food which is lovely, but by the chef/proprietor; Ugar Vata. He is just the most amazing host and, being in the service industry myself, I love the way he makes every diner feel so special. He greeted us on Friday night like long lost family, remembered so much about us including the fact that I love crème brulee and made the evening that much more memorable by the way he looked after us. I aspire to re-create his service ethos in our spas and health clubs and it was good to be reminded of what we are working towards.

Three: The final reason to be cheerful this week is that I know the smoke detectors in our house and the remote monitoring service are working just fine. The reason that I can say this with such certainty is that this morning I got a call whilst enjoying my coffee at The Forge from my father-in-law, Andrew, who was back at our house on his own to say the fire alarm was sounding. I promised him we would be back shortly . . . . and he assured me that he wasn't on fire! Moments later my mobile went again and it was the monitoring station explaining that the alarms were sounding and, as nobody had answered the phone at the house they had called the fire brigade who were on their way to the house! We raced back and got home just before the fire brigade arrived and it transpired that the cause of the alarm was father-in-law ironing directly under the smoke detector and being a little heavy with the steam obviously. Needless to say the fire officer wanted to check around the house fully to make sure we hadn't missed anything before admitting there was a first time for everything and that in his 15 year career he had never been called out before due to a man being over-zealous with an iron!

Never one to miss an opportunity, whilst the house was being checked, Andrew had taken Rose out to the fire engine and got her on the machine itself to take a few pictures. Her Mum, who was playing the cello this morning and so had to stay back at church for the second service was green with envy to have missed out on men in uniform visiting the house!

I think the fire officer took the whole thing in relatively good spirits and how can I have any complaints with Andrew given that he was home alone doing my ironing. The man is a legend!

So that's this weeks update. Tomorrow Miranda is back for more chemo and she also has a further scan on Wednesday to try to pin down why she has been struggling with shortness of breath over the past week. It is fair to say that her "good" week of last week hasn't been quite as good as normal. The shortness of breath problem has been coupled with blood tests showing that she is low on iron which could explain the tiredness she has also struggled with of late. This could lead to more medication, which given the number of tablets she is already taking no longer seems to phase her! We're halfway through the first stage of the treatment programme, three chemo injections gone and three more to go. It's a long journey but we are well on our way—thanks for making it this far with us.

19

Do You Really Mean That?

Its funny how there always seems to be something that crops up when I am least expecting it, to inspire or create the idea for my post, and this week is no different. But before I tell you about that I'm afraid there is something I need to confess. You see last night, on my way back from work, I stopped off at someone else's house. I had a cup of tea and as we sat around a table I looked into this rather beautiful girl's eyes and told her I loved her, with real meaning in my voice. And she looked into my eyes and told me that I was the best thing that had ever happened to her, and that she wanted to help me be the best I could possibly be. And then we kissed . . . .

Now before you get really angry with me and start thinking this is the most bizarre, cruellest way that anyone has admitted to an affair, let me explain that I'm part of the drama team at the Forge and last night was a practice for a sketch we are soon to perform. And despite the fact that Helen (or Liz as she is in the sketch!) seemed to really mean it when she said I'm the best thing to have happened to her; I'm not sure she really did mean it.

Isn't that sometimes true in real life also? Aren't we all guilty sometimes of saying things we don't really mean or maybe not backing up our words with actions?

(By the way I expect it will be about now that the colour will start to come back to my father-in-law's face if he has continued to read this far!!)

At the start of this week I had to speak at a Spa Conference in London and I was introduced as the MD from Imagine Spas who "have achieved so much with so little!" I wasn't quite sure how to take that comment but the conference host went on to explain that, although our spas weren't big in comparison to many others, when she had experienced them she found that we delivered great service with treatments that compared with the best. It was a lovely compliment and encouraged me. It reflects well on the teams and therapists in our spas and best of all, it means that, from the perspective of this one industry expert who introduced my talk, we deliver what we promise in our marketing. Our teams' actions back up the words and promises we make. I think that's really cool to be honest. But it has challenged and reminded me that we must never lose focus on that aspect of what we do.

But enough of my work—this is supposed to be all about how we cope with Miranda's illness. This week she has had her 4th chemo treatment and by now the cumulative effect of these treatments is starting to take its toll. She has also had a scan on her lung as her breathlessness was causing concern about the possibility of a blood clot, but fortunately that came back clear. She has felt really wiped out to be honest. Not in the way she did initially with the fever and hospital visits but just completely drained. Tonight I was back from London too late to put the children to bed and, wisely, Miranda asked a friend to come over to do that for her as she was just not up to it. Admitting to that fact is a sure sign of just how rough she feels!

The events of this week have made me think about what I say in these blogs and to friends. I can talk about how supportive I am but do I really back that up with actions? Does what I do, rather than what I say, make Miranda feel truly supported? Challenging thought that! Maybe I should finish this blog right now and go and tidy the kitchen, wash up and empty the dishwasher!

But before I do let me just explain what initially inspired this blog. When Miranda had her scan she was injected with some liquid which makes her slightly radio-active and she is not allowed near the children. It meant that I got to leave work early and pick the girls up from some friends who had looked after them. I had to take them home and do bathtime and bedtime by myself. Just before bed Rose handed me an envelope with my name on—"This is for you Daddy" she announced. I opened it up to find a card she had made from a craft set she had got for Christmas. I know I'm biased but, given she is only 5, it actually was quite impressive. Cut out using her serrated edged scissors and with colour and stripes and a few stickers it was . . . . well . . . . arty! Inside it said "To Daddy Love Rose" and there were lots of kisses. It is a source of embarrassment for me to admit that her writing is already more legible and neater than mine. It was very clear that an awful lot of time and effort had gone into making this card.

"What's this for" I asked her.

"Oh no reason Daddy," she said, "it's just because I love you"

My heart melted right there on the spot.

The thing is—it was the effort that had gone into the card that made it so special. The action backed up the words. I've put it on my desk at work—of course it's there to remind me of Rose but it is also there to remind me that what we say is nowhere near as important as what we do.

Amazing really—being taught a lesson in life by your five year old daughter.

I'm off to empty the dishwasher and I really do mean that! Oh and what about you? What do you need to do right now?

20

Follow the Signposts

I went for a run on Monday morning—nothing momentous in that, I know, but I had no planned route as I was on unfamiliar territory. I was staying away at a new residential spa in Essex called the Lifehouse—I'd gone there with my business partner for 24 hours to see what it had to offer and to do some business planning without the usual distractions of day-to-day work. It worked by the way—we got some useful stuff planned and the Lifehouse is very impressive.

Anyway back to my run. I have a reasonable sense of direction and a theory that if you keep turning right at every opportunity you soon end up where you started. So I set off with a determination to run for about 20 minutes. It was a beautiful morning—sun shining but there had been a sharp frost—so the trees and ground were wrapped in a silvery blanket that added a brightness and freshness to lift your spirit. Whether I got carried away enjoying the environment around me or whether I simply didn't turn right early enough I'm not sure but basically I got lost. Eventually I found a road and decided to maintain my "always turn right" theory expecting (desperately hoping in fact!) that this was the road out of the nearest village and towards the spa resort. Wrong again! I discovered I was actually running into the village on a totally different road to the one which led to the spa.

By the time I reached the village centre I had been running for about 30 minutes and was tired. Very tired. It would be fair to say that my run was laboured and my speed had dropped. There is nothing more embarrassing than being out for a run and being overtaken by a small 7 year old child walking to school . . . . with their Mum . . . . pushing a pushchair! I realised I was probably breathing heavily when women were crossing the road unnerved by my gasping for air behind them!

The only good thing about being in the village was that I was able to find road signs for the Lifehouse, could follow them, and get back on track and subsequently made it back to the spa. Suddenly running became easier again when I knew where I was going and was on the right path.

It made me think—isn't life a bit like that too?

This has been probably Miranda's toughest week since she started chemotherapy. The cumulative effect of the doses has kicked in with a vengeance and she has been totally wiped out, devoid of any energy plus the usual side effects of horrible taste, shortness of breath and irregular heartbeats. Last weekend she spent the vast majority of the time in bed on Saturday and, aside from insisting on cooking lunch, on Sunday was parked on the sofa. She found this incredibly frustrating and, understandably, it really got to her.

It made for a full on weekend for me too with sole responsibility for the children, getting to activities such as ballet and Church, washing to be done and getting the house tidy for the week etc. Rose and Millie found it difficult too as they love spending time with their Mum and this weekend it wasn't really an option. Millie is also at the age where tantrums are regular (hers not mine I mean!) and her favourite phrase is "I'll do it myself".

Whilst wanting to nurture and encourage her independence when "I'll do it myself" extends to zipping up her coat when we are already late for ballet this borders on exasperating. The choice is to either insist on zipping up the coat myself which will result in a meltdown screaming fit, or wait the extra 5 minutes it takes for Millie to do up the zip herself and be even more late!

Anyway I was doing fine until Sunday afternoon when my "patience tanks" were empty and Miranda made some inane comment which for some reason annoyed me and I got cross. Harsh words were spoken by me and I may even have raised my voice. Basically I got "lost", I was in unfamiliar territory. Here was my wife feeling at her worst thanks to her chemotherapy and I was getting ratty with her. I went back into the kitchen, washed up with a bit more vigour than was necessary and felt terrible. I tried to work out how I'd let myself get into that position and, more importantly, how I got back on track. I saw a sign we have hanging on the dresser in our kitchen that says "Live Well, Love Much, Laugh Often". I hadn't really done any of those things that day.

I think that in life, just like any other journey, we need "signposts" to follow. For me, those signposts often come from my faith. Irrespective of an individual's views on the whole "God thing" I'd challenge anyone to argue that the signposts, the way to live life, as taught through the stories of the Bible are not a good way to live.

Inevitably there are going to be times in life when, just like on that run on Monday, I'm going to lose my way, be on unfamiliar territory. And what is going to count, is not how many times I get into that position, but how quickly I look out for the right signposts and how diligently I then follow them. The past week has taught me that, while we journey awhile with cancer, I need to be a bit more focussed on the road ahead and on following those signposts! And if I do that—it will all seem so much easier.

So if you should bump into me and I'm looking a bit hot and bothered and my breathing is heavy, feel free to point me in the right direction won't you. Please. I will be very grateful.

21

Burst Out the Prison

Last Friday I went back to Leeds to my old college, Carnegie, for a tribute dinner for a former lecturer Wilf Paish who passed away in January of last year. Over 300 people were at the dinner which is testament to Wilf's popularity and, in a fitting tribute, a large sum of money was raised to create a legacy in Wilf's name that will help disadvantaged children develop their sporting talent. I think Wilf would have loved that.

It was a great night, I went with Steve Taylor, my business partner who I met at Carnegie, and Ian Wakefield who is one of my best and longest standing friends. I gave Ian his first job in health and fitness when he was 17 and he's now Business Development Manager for the newly formed Institute for Management of Sport and Physical Activity, the lead body for the industry. Wilf had coached Ian at the javelin. The evening was capped off with a tribute from the legendary Tom McNab, an incredible coach in his own right, who also wrote the best seller, Flanagans Run, which was turned into a Disney film and was Technical Advisor to the film Chariots of Fire. Tom is a great speaker and his memories of Wilf lit up the room.

After a great catch up over breakfast the next morning with Ian in Starbucks on the Otley Road and a chance to see all my old college haunts I headed back home. As I drove down the A1 I had time to think about Wilf and what he had achieved and the impact he had made on me. Longer than expected in fact as roadworks added over an hour to my journey!

You see Wilf will probably be best remembered for the fact that he coached Tessa Sanderson to Olympic Gold at the Los Angeles Olympics. A victory achieved against the odds beating rivals who were much more fancied for Gold. He also coached Peter Elliott to an equally unexpected Silver at the Seoul Olympics and worked for many years with Mick Hill, a leading javelin thrower. He was a brilliant coach for elite athletes but that is such a small part of the incredible man that he was.

His understanding of sporting skills and techniques was matched by his incredible knowledge of anatomy, physiology and biomechanics. As my lecturer in those subjects he brought them alive in a way that no one else could. He nurtured my desire to understand how the human body works and the knowledge I gained from him underpinned my confidence to work in health clubs and start Fitness Express with Steve.

He broke down complicated techniques and moves and made it so simple. His analysis of all the throwing disciplines in athletics was simple:

"Chin, knee, toe; make a bow; see it go"

And he was right, look at any of javelin, shot putt etc and you will see the athlete starts with their chin, knee and toe in line, puts their body into a bow shape and then releases the implement as they uncoil. So simple and yet so memorable.

But to talk about his amazing knowledge of the technical aspects still doesn't do justice to who Wilf was. He also recognised the importance of passion and commitment and desire over natural ability. He was an incredible motivator; in fact I would go as far as saying he was the most motivational person I have met.

Wilf understood that to be successful you needed natural ability. Small in stature, he would often claim—"I would have been Olympic Champion at the High Jump if I had chosen my parents more carefully". But he also knew that you needed an inner desire, commitment and passion to go with that natural ability. Wilf loved the underdog and you can see that through the people he chose to coach at elite level, many of whom over-achieved against expectation.

But it wasn't just the elite athlete that Wilf enjoyed coaching. He was often at his happiest coaching at grass roots level. He loved spotting potential in people. I had the joy of organising some health and fitness short break holidays with Wilf at a holiday centre in Suffolk I worked in whilst at university and beyond. I saw him coach people who were keen but not necessarily gifted. And I saw him spot something in them that often, the individual themselves didn't know they had. I saw the joy in their faces as Wilf teased this ability out of them. The fun and laughter he brought was just wonderful to experience.

His humour and sense of fun was also something that I connected with. At Carnegie the PA to the Head of School, had a dog which she sometimes had to bring to the office. It sat in a basket in the corner of the office. Wilf decided that from a physiology perspective the dog should be able to high jump and over a period of a few weeks he got the dog to perform a high jump. Needless to say, over time, he also got the dog to improve too!

A story about Wilf that Tom McNab told in his tribute speech particularly resonated with me. I remembered Wilf telling it to me too. Wilf taught about how we all have a tendency to live within the walls of our own self-imposed limits in what we believe we can achieve. We all frame what we believe we can do and, more importantly, what we believe is beyond us. Wilf passionately believed that it was these walls that became a prison cell to our true potential. He told how to reach what we were really capable of we need to "burst out of the prison"—to believe that we can succeed against all the odds and to just keep reaching for the next level. He told it far more powerfully than I can convey here but it has had an impact on me throughout my life and especially in developing Fitness Express with Steve. I came to realise that Wilf was so right.

And as I drove down the A1 I also thought about my wife and her battle with cancer. I thought about her incredible determination, about how so many people keep telling me how well she looks and how little impact the chemo seems to be having on her everyday life. I thought about how from day one she has never doubted that she will get through this, how the cancer means just a course of treatment and when that is over, it is over. I thought about how she is actively planning our garden, booking herself on a course so that she can build us our own outdoor pizza oven. She has well and truly "burst out the prison" that a cancer diagnosis might so easily put any of us in.

Literally as I have been writing this blog it has just been announced that Erik Abidal, the Barcelona full back has been diagnosed with liver cancer. Only last week I watched him play a great game against Arsenal in the Champions League. It is one more reminder that this horrible disease can strike anyone at anytime. Now cancer is part of my everyday life, such news has a different effect on me than before. Of course there is still the sense of shock and disbelief. Erik is only 31, my wife is 36. But now I have a perspective on how he, and more directly, his immediate family will be feeling—the numbness, the disbelief, the fear, the sense of entering an unknown. May they find a way to "burst out the prison" too.

Wilf never met my wife but I think he would have liked her. He would have admired her determination and her spirit. I can imagine him saying to her something like:

"C'mon luv, you'll beat this thing for sure. You'll beat it because you know you can".

And he would be right of course.

There was a lot of talk on Friday night about Wilf's legacy. Many people spoke about the true legacy of the man being the effect he had on the many people he coached and taught and I think that is so true. He's left an indelible footprint on my life and I will do all I can to keep tearing down the walls that limit what I think I can do. After all that Wilf has taught me it's the least I can do. He demanded and deserves nothing less.

Thanks Wilf.

22

Unforgettable

So last Sunday Miranda was feeling much better and we headed off to Aldeburgh after the usual trip to the Forge. Aldeburgh is one of my favourite places; typically Suffolk and a combination of lovely restaurants and shops whilst retaining much of the charm of a traditional fishing village. You can still walk along the beach and buy fresh fish from the many fishermen's huts that line the top of the beach. Or you can join the queue that snakes along the High Street for the legendary Fish and Chip shop which attracts visitors from far and wide. The wait to be served is worth it by the way. We had lunch at Prezzos, the girl's favourite restaurant, and then headed off to the Peter Pears Gallery to see "Unforgettable," an exhibition of almost 3oo paintings. Now I know that it sounds like we are asking for trouble taking a 5 year old and a 2 year old to an art exhibition but this one was a little different.

It was organised by Young Art East Anglia and was the culmination of a competition run in over 60 schools across the region with almost 2,000 paintings entered by children of primary school age. So whilst trying desperately hard not to sound too full of parental pride, the reason we went was because Rose's painting was one of the 300 winners that had been chosen to be exhibited. I have to say the standard of paintings was very good and there were many different interpretations of the theme of "Unforgettable". Holidays seemed to be a popular choice although the graphic depiction by one child of their first ever vaccination did particularly catch my eye! It was the blood dripping from the arm and the size of the needle in relation to their body that made me smile!

I'm not sure what the criteria was for judging but let's just say that Rose's painting was more allegorical than most and I think a beach was involved . . . . probably! I'm assuming the judge was into abstract art and chose Rose's as he saw something in it that, to be totally honest, was lost on me! Good job that an interview with each artist was not involved as I asked Rose if she could explain what the rather dramatic swirls in the middle of her painting were—"no idea Daddy" was her reply!

Clearly I'm only jealous that at the age of five she has achieved something—having her artwork exhibited at one of Suffolk's leading galleries—which I have failed to achieve in forty-five years! Her art skills must come from her mother. I remember that Art at school was the one subject that I never got better than a "C" grade for any work submitted. Indeed I always remember one of the best comments I got on any art homework was "a reasonably good effort in its own rather inaccurate way". It was a very fair assessment and made me a little proud of it to be honest. Funny how some school memories just stick with you!

In one of those weird, quirky moments that life throws at you, the whole Young Art East Anglia event was run in aid of Cancer Research UK and there was a moment when I did wonder if Rose had slipped through on the sympathy vote. However a quick check confirmed that entries were submitted and judging had taken place prior to Miranda's diagnosis so clearly I was being very unfair on her.

All the winners had their paintings printed up onto postcards and so we bought the entire remaining stock of Rose's effort and Miranda has spent the last few days posting them on to Grandparents and Auntie Lou etc.

After the exhibition we went down to the beach. The tide was in so the beach was just pebbles and we stood for a while and threw stones in the sea. Why is that just the most compelling, but strangely comforting thing to do? Then we bumped into our friends, Chris and Jane, and chatted for a while before the girls and me chased each other around the beach and tried to put stones down each other's back. Squeals of delight rang out in the air—and the girls were laughing a bit too!

Miranda was feeling a bit tired so went and sat on a bench by a fisherman's hut and watched as we continued to play. It is so tough for her not being able to join in as normal but that's the impact of the chemo unfortunately. With Millie the excitement and laughter is greatest when she senses I'm about to catch her. Her sense of fun is infectious. Eventually the three of us were too tired to run anymore so we laid down on the beach and Rose decided that she and Millie would try to bury me under stones. They gave it a go for a while although they ended up with lots of stones on them too!

And then the sun came out briefly and the three of us just lay there looking up at the blue sky and we talked a little. We spotted the vapour trails of a plane flying very high overhead. I told them that in that tiny dot of a plane which we could see would probably be around 200 people.

"Wow", said Rose, "where is it going to Daddy?"

"No idea—where do you think it's going?" I asked.

"Disneyland" said Rose.

"The Moon" suggested Millie.

We laughed a lot. We counted seagulls that flew overhead and gave them all names—Cyril was our favourite. I had my arms around them and I told them both how much I loved them and then we just lay there for a while, not saying anything, just staring up at this big, beautiful, blue sky with wispy, white swirls of cloud gently ambling from left to right. And I thought how outrageously fortunate I am to get to live this life. Sure there are bits of it that are pretty rubbish and it's fair to say that as a family we are getting our fair share of tough moments right now. But when you remember the freedom we have to run on a beach, to throw stones, to laugh, to enjoy being with each other or to just lie back and soak up the beauty of nature around us. I mean it's pretty amazing don't you think?

Unforgettable in fact.

23

TGI Friday

This has been one of those weeks where somehow just getting to Friday night seems an achievement in its own right! That might sound a bit pathetic I know but this has definitely been a challenging week!

Monday was the day Miranda was due her fifth round of chemotherapy. We had agreed with the school that we would take Rose along with us as she had been keen to understand what happened when her Mum went for her "special medicine". So the three of us trooped off to the hospital and were settling in to the chemo club lounge when news came through that for the first time Miranda's white blood cell count was too low to allow them to give her the chemotherapy treatment. This was a bit of blow and a problem that we had not encountered before. It was tough on Miranda who had psyched herself up for the treatment and was now faced with a 48 hour delay. Rose was disappointed to have missed out supporting her Mum through the process and I was left to rearrange a full day of meetings on the Wednesday and try to work out how I crammed 5 days work into 3 days! As I write this on the Friday night it doesn't feel like I've done a very good job in that regard to be honest. We had a consultation with the oncologist and then headed home mid-afternoon with a sense of a wasted day. And it was my birthday too!

Anyway onto Wednesday and Miranda's blood count had risen enough to just get over the level required and we were on for the treatment. This problem with her white blood count was a useful reminder for Miranda of the need to take things easier and treat this whole programme with a bit of respect. Since the challenges of the first dose which sent her neutropenic and into hospital she has been able to avoid any such problems with later doses thanks largely to a "magic bullet" injection 24 hours after chemo is administered. By her own admission this has meant she has been a bit blasé about allowing her body time to recover in her "good" week and has, naturally, tried to cram as much as she can in to the time when she feels vaguely OK. Lesson learnt!

The treatment went relatively straight forward and by moving to Wednesday we got to meet a completely different group of people who form the Chemo Club Crew for Wednesday. They are a lively lot it is fair to say and when this included making Easter bonnets out of upturned cardboard vomit bowls, decorated with coffee stirrers and consultation cards cut into the shape of tulip petals I knew I was out of my depth! Any suggestions as to how I compete in three weeks time when we will join them again would be much appreciated!

We got home in time to go to Rose's school for what was my first parents evening and it was so encouraging to hear how well she is doing and we got to see her workbooks. I loved reading through her work and was touched to see that when they had to write a letter to someone explaining about their Christmas activities Rose had chosen to write to her late Grandpa (my Dad).

"Dear Grandpa, We are sorry you couldn't be with us this Christmas . . . ." was how she had started the letter. Me too Rose, I thought as I found a lump had arrived suddenly in my throat!

We chatted with her teacher, Mrs Burgess, about Miranda's illness and how Rose was dealing with it at school. We were told that Rose seems to have taken it in her stride and talks about her Mum's cancer in a matter of fact way. We were so encouraged that Mrs Burgess felt we were doing the right thing by being open with Rose and including her in what is happening. All very reassuring and once more I found myself being hugely proud of my eldest daughter.

But the day's excitement did not end there. We arrived home to the sound of crying from upstairs and Rose stationed by the back door saying that Mummy had to go straight up to the bathroom. It transpired that whilst both girls were having a bath supervised by Grandma, Millie had suddenly had a fit which lasted a couple of minutes. It appears that Grandma had once more been brilliant getting Millie out of the bath and putting her into the recovery position and gently wiping the foam from her mouth with a towel.

Clearly I think this was a shameless and basic attempt by Millie to divert the attention away from her mother. It worked to be fair. A trip back to the hospital—this time to A&E ensued for Miranda, Millie and Grandma whilst I stayed at home with a distraught Rose. She was clearly very worried about her sister and was eventually persuaded that it was best for her to go to bed rather than wait up. I agreed to put a picture of Millie on the wall by Rose's bed so that she could still see her and think about her. Rose does have a compassionate nature.

I paced the house waiting for news which came through to report that Millie had been diagnosed with tonsillitis and that the "fit" was a febrile convulsion which is common in very young children when their temperature spikes apparently. Sighs of relief all round. The tonsillitis has made Millie quite poorly and whilst writing this blog we have had to go up to her as she has been sick in her bed. This is not good news and I have got my wellies out in case she continues to be sick through the night!

The cumulative effect of the chemo is also kicking in now and Miranda is starting to feel fairly ropey so a quiet weekend is planned. I will be trying to be as good a nurse as I can be to both Millie and Miranda over the next couple of days before a rested Grandma rides back in to the rescue on Sunday night. That woman is a lifesaver!

As I put Rose to bed tonight we contemplated how lucky we were to both be feeling fit and healthy although we did wonder if we could drum up any sympathy for the tiny graze Rose obtained on her knee in the school playground and the small paper cut I have on my little finger. What do you think? No chance? Really? Oh well we will soldier on I suppose. It is Friday after all!

24

Keep Your Hair On

Can I just say that as I write this blog I am aware that compared to many other people I realise I am in such a fortunate position. Only today I learnt of a former employee who has just lost his only daughter at the age of 12. I have no idea how you begin to come to terms with that. I simply need to turn on the TV to see what is happening in other parts of the world such as Japan and the Middle East to realise that my day to day existence is a relative walk in the park. I think it is really important to keep a little perspective in place at times such as these.

So in the context of that introduction I want to just tell you a bit about our week so far.

We are now developing a new kind of code in our house. If Miranda is feeling really, really rough with the chemo then she doesn't wear her wig. She knows that she won't be going out or seeing anyone and on bad days can't bear the tightness of the wig on her head. She shuffles around the house in a sweat top with the hood up. It's like living with a teenage hoodie with the attitude to match! I have to say that if the roles were reversed and I had this horrible disease with its debilitating side effects I would be far more grouchy and miserable than Miranda is. No doubt about it. And I understand her sheer frustration at not having the energy or ability to do the most basic of activities. On her really bad days that frustration gets worked out on me, her Mum and to a lesser extent the children and we have generally coped with it fairly well providing everything else is on an even keel.

Unfortunately this past week the arrival of the teenage hoodie for a couple of days coincided with Millie being poorly with tonsillitis. It meant that Miranda and Millie spent most of their time cuddling up on the sofa watching TV whilst Rose and I got on with the weekend as best we could. Rose was just about OK with this but there was a bit of jealousy that Millie dominated all the time with her Mum and was also not interested in playing with Rose. It's been tough on Rose and once the weekend was over and my workload meant she didn't get to see me at all either, she has struggled. There has been the odd sign for a while that she is finding it harder to deal with her Mum's illness but yesterday Rose got a pencil and drew on the sitting room carpet. It is a really perturbing thing for her to have done.

We had been warned that often children dealt with this illness in a parent by showing some regressive behaviour but seeing as she never did this type of thing at the age of 2 it is slightly alarming and so out of character as she is just a few months shy of her 6th birthday. A trip to the family support officer from the MacMillan Trust at the hospital is being arranged for Miranda and I so that we can see if there is anything more we could, or should, be doing to help Rose through this. And then we probably need to call into Carpet World on the way home too!

Whilst this is obviously a horrible time for Miranda, I think the hardest thing for the rest of us to deal with is the complete sense of helplessness. The sense of standing by and just watching Miranda struggling so much without being able to do anything is so difficult. Each time I watch her, well it just bruises my soul. And it hurts. Really hurts. And I just hate the impact it has on my children too.

On the flip side, her indomitable spirit is an inspiration. She got her hair back on yesterday and went off for a day's training in growing cut flowers. It's left her tired but she loved it and has come back full of ideas and plans. Tonight she has been showing me all the flowers she intends to grow in the various beds, borders and tubs in our garden. She is amazing!

So that's our week—it is ending better than it started that's for sure. I will be putting up another post on Sunday in celebration of Mothers Day and reflecting on what I've learnt about being a son and a parent. Then you can also look out for a second entry on the blog from Miranda which she is currently writing and hopes to post up next week! I've had a sneak preview and it's a good one!

Meanwhile the main hope here, as we head into the weekend, is that Miranda keeps her hair on!

25

Letter to My Mother

When Miranda was diagnosed with cancer just before Christmas I mentally went through the family and tried to imagine how each of them would deal with the situation. In almost every case I have been surprised at how well everyone, including me(!), has coped with it. However the one exception which I didn't anticipate is the difficulty my Mum has had dealing with the situation. I think this is largely due to the fact that she naturally wants to help, needs to feel wanted and yet we are not really able to cope with her and all the challenges that Miranda's illness brings. This has led to some upset and tension which has been an unwanted and frustrating sideshow over the past few months to be totally honest. It has given me cause to reflect on the role of parents and how we interact with our children. So in an attempt to try to explain how I feel and to recognise all that my Mum has done for me over the past 46 years I have written a letter to accompany her Mothers Day card.

I have always tried to be completely honest through this blog and so I've decided to post up the letter to my Mum as it reflects how I'm feeling right now and, more importantly, what I've learnt about relationships with our parents and with our children. Of course I'm not expecting that everyone will agree with me and I'm sure as I get older and wiser my views will change as experience is the best possible teacher.

Thanks again for travelling with me on this journey and a Happy Mothers Day to all Mums reading this—you really are very special people.

Dear Mum

Happy Mothers Day! I thought it was worth putting a few reflections down on paper as the last 4 months have been tough on all of us.

I want you to know that I really love you and that I think you are a really wonderful Mum, not least, because you are my Mum. I realise how difficult you have found dealing with the situation we find ourselves in with Miranda's illness and that, at times, you've felt excluded from what is going on and a bit helpless. I'm sorry that's the case.

Before I go on to say why I think that has happened I want to just talk you through what I've learnt so far in the five and a half years I've been a Dad. You see I'd never felt any real affinity with babies and whenever I've been introduced to a friend's new arrival and given the baby to hold I've always tried to assess what the minimum time is that I can hold their little "bundle of joy" without offending them by handing it back! So when Miranda was pregnant I really worried that it would be a few years before I felt any affection or bond with my, soon to arrive, son or daughter.

It was pointless worrying. When Rose was born it was like God opened up this new chamber in my heart, with a volume akin to the Royal Albert Hall, and filled it to bursting point with love for this tiny baby in my arms. It was overwhelming. I realised in an instant that there was nothing Rose could do to make me love her any more and nothing she could do to make me love her any less. It was the first time I truly understood what unconditional love really meant. A powerful and incredible emotion.

I came home and wrote Rose a card which I presented her with when, after 3 days, she arrived home for the first time—this is what it said:

"Dear Rose

Welcome home darling!

I just want you to know that your Mum and I will do everything we can to make this place as full of laughter and love as the home that I grew up in with Nanny and Grandpa and that your Mum grew up in with Grandma and Granddad and Aunty Lou.

I cannot describe just how proud and happy I am to have you as my daughter. Mum and I will do everything we can to help you learn what is important in life and what isn't.

Please be assured that for the rest of our lives our home will be somewhere that you will be loved completely and unconditionally, and where a hug is always available at anytime day or night.

With all my love forever
Dad x"

At the time that seemed to me to sum up what my role as a Dad was all about. And to be honest that view has still not changed. I remember reading it to Rose when she got home and I think I secretly hoped she would be so moved by it that she would defy all laws of maturity and at 3 days old throw her little arms around me, speak her first words along the lines of "crickey Dad 3 days in and you are already a legend to me"!

In reality she looked vaguely in my direction, puckered her lips a little, gurgled and I felt the warmth of baby sick run down my arm but fortunately not onto the card! We've kept the card of course and one day I hope Rose may see it and treasure it but I rather suspect it will always have far more meaning for me than it does for her.

It was about five days later and still finding myself overwhelmed by love for Rose when it suddenly dawned on me. The love I have for Rose, the hopes, dreams and fears about her future—it's exactly the same as you and Dad had for me. It's pretty obvious I suppose but I'd never thought of it in that way before. I then spooled through my life and all the things I'd done and said and how hard so much of that must have been for you. I was imagining Rose doing those same things and how I would feel. I was horrified. I remember calling you and Dad to apologise. Believe me—it was the most heartfelt apology I've ever made!

I've now realised that parenting is the most challenging and rewarding role that any of us ever have. It is often a thankless task but just a smile and the word "Daddy" can make it all so worthwhile. Right now Rose and Millie need and want me to do everything for them; get them dressed, put them to bed, carry them around, read them stories, play with them, wipe their bottoms, everything. And I do all of it willingly and lovingly and dread the time when I don't get to do that anymore, well maybe I'll be happy to stop wiping their bottoms but you get my drift. Every single time when I'm held up with work and miss putting them to bed, I'm driving back thinking to myself well that is one bedtime story that I will never get back, one less night I will get to read to them.

At the weekends, after breakfast, Rose, Millie and I go upstairs and clean our teeth together and I put mousse my hair. One of them gets the jar out of the cupboard and we make a joke about the old advert that went "there's a mousse loose about this hoose!" We laugh every time. However, I know that all too soon, I will be going upstairs on my own to do those things. I'm sad even now at just the thought of that. But that's the thing with parenting, our role is to prepare our children for the life that lies ahead, to teach them to stand on their own two feet, to gain independence, live their own life and be the people they were created to be. The challenge is every step they take towards that independence requires us, as parents, to give up something we had loved doing with them. Boy oh boy, Rose is only five and I'm finding this challenging whatever will I be like when she's fifteen?!

I've also learnt that the role of a Mum and Dad is very different. Miranda's illness has meant that I get to take Rose to ballet 2 out of 3 Saturdays. For Rose, ballet is something she wants to do with her Mum—every time I take her there are tears, last-minute phantom illnesses to try to get out of going. It's hard work persuading her to go. I really want her to enjoy going to ballet with me but she never will. So rather than get upset at the things I can't share with Rose I have learnt to find things that she loves doing with me and focus on doing those as often as we can. I can't be her Mum, I've just got to be her Dad. And for Rose and Millie I am so determined to be the best Dad I can be.

So all of this leads me to say, on this Mothers Day, thank you for being the best Mum to me that you could be. Thank you for the way that you have supported me in the things I have done, for encouraging me and for challenging me when you felt it necessary, even though I may not have appreciated that at the time. You devoted so much time to me and never for one moment in my life have I questioned or doubted your love for me. I believe that certainty of being loved is the single most powerful thing any parent can give their child.

Thank you for sitting with me for hours on end at night when as a young child I couldn't get to sleep and was scared of being on my own. Thank you for all the honest and real and deep conversations we'd often have about life when I got home from school over cup of tea before I tackled my homework. I could never have had that level of conversation with Dad and although we often disagreed the process of debate you made me go through was so valuable. I treasure those memories. Thank you for modelling for me what it means to be generous—I've watched you help others in so many ways throughout my life and even now at 78 you continue to cook Sunday lunch for ladies who aren't able to do that for themselves. I admire that so much. And thank you so much for all the times throughout my life that you, and Dad, have cooked, cleaned, maintained and sorted the gardens out at the various houses I've lived in.

All those things you've done have shaped me into the person I am now. I hope that I can be as diligent and dedicated in this regard with Rose and Millie as you and Dad have been with me.

So even though you helped prepare me for it, I guess it is still tough watching me going through this period of time with Miranda's cancer. If you are really honest, it must be difficult not to feel left out with Barbara, Miranda's Mum, spending so much time at our house to help us.

However, the simple fact is that all our focus now has to be with Miranda. Aside from the fact that Barbara is well over 10 years younger than you and therefore more able to cope with the workload we heap on her, she is also Miranda's Mum, and when you feel really rough and life is pretty rubbish there is no substitute for having your Mum around. I think also that having to watch your youngest daughter battle a life threatening illness must be just about the worst possible experience any parent can go through. So I am sure that immersing herself in providing such practical help is really helping Barbara to get through this time too.

I realise that the way you are wired up is to provide help to others. I think that is in your DNA. It is through helping people that you have a sense of purpose and value. I know that part of the trauma of losing Dad is that over the last few years of his life he relied on you so much that you felt valued in providing that practical support to him. With his passing not only went the love of your life but that sense of value and purpose too. No wonder it has been difficult to come to terms with.

But having said all that, right now, we need to get through this in the way that we are doing and the practical support we need comes from Barbara and our friends nearby. That is in no way a poor reflection on you it is just how it needs to be.

So after a lifetime of helping me in so many practical ways you are free to play with the grandchildren, encourage, support and cheer on but, for a change, not have to "do". I hope you understand and that you can accept that position with a level of empathy for how Barbara and Miranda must be feeling right now.

Once again I need you to understand and I need you to let go, this time, of the desire to help out. As I'm fast learning, as a parent, letting go is a key requirement and yet it is the toughest thing to do.

Happy Mother's Day
All my love
Dave x

26

In My Line of Vision
(Miranda's Second Post)

It's nearly three months since Miranda wrote her first post on this blog and as she approaches the finishing straight of chemotherapy and our thoughts turn to the next stage of the treatment programme we felt it was high time she let you know how she is feeling. Once more, I think you will find her writing a powerful and insightful read. And naturally I just want to remind you all that I am so immensely proud of her . . . .

In My Line of Vision

Something dawned on me last week as I was watching the news. I was actually reminded how small I am (and I don't mean in a vertically-challenged kind of a way!) and how really very fortunate I am. Here am I faced with, what to me, is a major health problem, which impacts me directly and naturally has a knock-on effect on those closest to me. There is also a bit of a ripple effect touching our friends and acquaintances, having more impact on some than on others. Stop and consider the Japan earthquake and tsunami, and the hugely devastating immediate impact on lives, buildings and land. And the ripple effect of that is enormous, and effects of it will be felt by thousands of people for years to come be it through loss, grief, injury, radiation and more. That really puts my life into perspective—if my illness were an earthquake, it would barely figure on the Richter Scale.

Later on in the news, another story caught my attention. I don't know if you saw it, or have seen the story in the papers regarding breast cancer prevention drugs? Cancer experts are hoping to prescribe preventative drugs to women in high-risk categories of developing breast cancer. What dawned on me as the story went on was that I wouldn't find myself in the high-risk category, and therefore even if preventative drugs were already available, I believe it is highly unlikely that I would have been pinpointed to receive them.

I remember when we met with the breast consultant back in December for the diagnosis, her words were, "You've just been really unlucky". So true!

Now I don't profess to being a "green" Goddess by any means, but I try to ensure we do what we can to live a life that is reasonably well in tune with our environment; I am conscious about the chemicals that are found in the food we eat and products we use and aim to avoid these as much as possible; I had about a 20 year spell of eating no meat (I succumbed for practical reasons in January 2010), and now I am still very particular about it being "happy" meat; I keep fairly fit (organised exercise may have dropped to one session a week but the children keep me fit!); I think we eat fairly well; I am not obese, or overweight, nor do I smoke, I don't drink (excessively); I like to consider myself as still being in the 'young' category (though unfortunately I do just fall into the 36-45 age group when form-filling!); I breastfed both my girls for at least the first 6 months of their lives; and there is no family history of breast cancer in my family. I will spare you unnecessary detail but neither were my breasts particularly dense! Breast Cancer? Unlucky? I should say so!!

The other thing that is beginning to sink is the fact that, according to Cancer Research UK, "almost two out of every three women with breast cancer survive for more than 20 years and more than three-quarters of women with breast cancer survive for at least 10 years". Maybe I have been naively optimistic over the last 3 or 4 months, as I am determined to keep focus on the treatment for what it is, but as I face an appointment with the breast consultant and my oncologist this week to discuss surgery and radiotherapy treatment, questions about prognosis are seeping in to the back of my mind.

In the moments when I am not feeling so strong, of course the questions enter my head: what if the treatment doesn't work? What if it comes back? What if I'm in the 25% of women who don't survive 10 years? I may not even see Millie reach high school. But, I can't let myself go there, because it's not helpful or productive in any way. Yes, there are times when I wish I could just run away and hide—I remember the first time I set foot in the Oncology department and saw people wearing scarves on their heads; had I not been holding tightly on to Dave's hand then, I would have run—but that wouldn't actually help anyone, least of all me, or my family. But I guess it would be unrealistic to expect I wouldn't have those thoughts at times.

I am reading a book at the moment by Wendy Bray, called "In the Palm of God's Hands", a diary of her diagnosis and treatment of Hodgkins Lymphoma, and subsequent breast cancer diagnosis. Wendy describes in her book that when you get given exclusive membership of the "cancer club", how suddenly you can feel no longer eligible for membership of any other "club" as you get forgotten and left behind by everyone else carrying on with their normal, busy everyday lives, or the treatment has made you too unwell, fat or unattractive to be included. When I read that, I actually thought how fortunate I am to have such wonderful friends, who make sure whether it be via text, Facebook, email, phone, letter, flowers, magazine subscription, a food parcel or running the Race for Life that we are still very much in their thoughts and that I'm still in the "club"!

I hope it doesn't sound too vain to say that I'm really relieved I haven't ballooned in weight or become unrecognisable as a result of the treatment because no matter what anyone says, it does matter what I look like, if for no other reason than for my own self-esteem. I may have yellowing, ridged nails and very little hair, but I still have eyebrows, eyelashes and my figure (more or less, but I can't blame the drugs for the extra bulges, rather it is down to too much comfort food and no exercise!)—thank you God for small mercies!

I think also because I don't look especially unwell, I struggle at times to accept the seriousness of my illness. I do believe however that there is a difference between being optimistic and having a positive outlook, and believing 100% that I am going to soon be told that I am completely better and cured. That, I think, would be naive. In 5 years time, I really hope to walk away from a consultant's appointment with the all-clear—it would be a shame at that point to leave the hospital and get hit by a bus, wouldn't it? But isn't that just it? None of us really has any idea how numbered our days might be, it's just that at the moment the question mark hangs just a little more within my line of vision.

So I do ask myself . . . Why did I push myself just a little bit (maybe too much?) last Wednesday to attend a cutting garden course to inspire me to fill our garden with colour?; why did I push myself just a little (too much again?) to attend the Mothers' Day lunch with Rose at her school?; why am I absolutely determined (health permitting—and rather frustratingly, at the moment, it is a nasty eye infection that might prevent me) to head back to Warwickshire next weekend to play in a concert and a chance to catch up with some really great friends and my parents?; why are we spending a weekend away with a fab group of friends in Norfolk at the end of April?; why am I dead-set on building a pizza oven in our garden this summer? That question mark I told you about . . . well, it's not going to obstruct my view so much that I don't see the opportunities to do the little things that really matter . . . even if it does take just a little bit more effort at the moment.

As I've learnt over the last few months—that extra bit of effort is always worth it.

27

Does My Tum Look Big Enough in This? (Miranda's Third Post)

At the risk of feeling that she is taking over my blog I've allowed Miranda to write another post to update on our latest hospital visit when I spent the morning sat in a room with 4 women looking at pictures of reconstructed breasts. I am still recovering! I feel the level of knowledge I now have on this subject is beyond that with which I am comfortable. I think my level of humour is such that any retelling of that morning's events could leave me in serious trouble and so here is the update of what we learnt and what is happening to Miranda as we approach the second stage of our journey. I will be back next week meanwhile those of a sensitive nature may want to look away now . . . !

It would appear it is my turn again; not quite sure whether that is a good thing or not, and hope you don't mind hearing from me again so soon. Due to the delicate nature of the subject, Dave felt it would be better for me to do this update, although I do feel I'm robbing him of the opportunity to make a few jokes . . . but maybe you'll agree with me and think that is probably a good thing?!

This week has included an appointment with the breast consultant, who I haven't seen since my diagnosis, and my oncologist . . . or so we thought. It turned out that the breast consultant was on holiday, which was frustrating to say the

102

least, as Dave had taken the day off work specially to come to this appointment with me, and we were hoping to get answers to questions and get lots of information about surgery and radiotherapy, and hopefully get dates in the diary as to when these would happen.

Dave made it known (in his very diplomatic yet strongly assertive business-like way! . . . I thought for a moment we were about to secure a deal on a new spa!) that he was rather disappointed about the absence of the breast consultant. This expression of dissatisfaction actually achieved a great result and saved us a trip to Chelmsford to have my fat assessed (more on that later), and we actually were rather glad in the end that the breast consultant hadn't been there! Funny how these things work out!

Anyway, I will do my best to keep this brief and keep the number of breast-related jokes to a minimum—oh, I feel out of my depth already, it really should be a man writing this! The next stage of this as you'll have gathered by now is surgery, which is likely to take place in the second week of May. The oncologist advised that only one mastectomy will be clinically necessary at this stage, which is a relief to hear—I wasn't looking forward to making the decision if they had said it was up to me to decide if I "wanted" to have both removed or not. The biggest issue, which may or may not involve a choice, is the type of reconstruction. Can I just say at this stage, that this conversation was pretty eye-opening and it left me amazed at what surgeons can do nowadays!

But if you wish you stop reading now, I won't be at all offended!

One option I have ruled out, as it brings with it a future of aches and pains following the operation, uses a flap of muscles and tissue brought round to the front from my back. The second option involves a silicon implant—they have however (fortunately!) come up with a new technique to ensure you get a natural 'droop', so I'm hopeful if I end up with this option that when I lie down, both breasts will dutifully fall south! Is this too much information? Do you really want to know all this? The third option involves a tummy tuck! Now many women might jump for joy at this suggestion. My problem is that I may not have enough tummy to make this possible! Now, before I get inundated with emails, I have already received several offers from friends offering to donate fat—whilst it is a very kind and generous offer, unfortunately I don't get the feeling that the consultants will be able to take you up on it, but thank you anyway! The disadvantage with this last option is that the operation takes several hours longer (as the fat has to removed carefully to ensure blood vessels survive—sadly not just a case of liposuction!) and the likely recovery time is several weeks longer than with the implant method due to the 8inch incision across my belly—worse than a caesarean!

I'm trying not to think about it too much at the moment, as I don't know at this stage whether or not I have an option—in the meantime I am eating as much as I possibly can in an attempt to fatten myself up a bit . . . never felt quite so much like a turkey before! We have an appointment on Monday with a consultant who will be able to say by looking at me whether I have enough fat on my tummy. I am really hoping that she thinks I have, or at least could have with a high calorie diet over the next 4 weeks, if for no other reason than to give me an option. Because you can be sure that if I don't have the option I'll want the option I can't have. It's quite ironic that I've spent most of my adult life exercising to stay slim, and now I'm wishing I was a bit fatter!

It was an appointment of mixed emotions; frustrating, disappointing, challenging, scary, daunting, and yet still had moments when I knew if I caught Dave's eye we would both giggle like little school children. Well so would you if someone suggested to you quite seriously that you could always have stick-on nipples if you didn't want to have another operation at a later date! And just the mention of 'support' groups in the context of breasts had both of us biting our tongues quite hard!

I'm conscious that is probably too much information, but you read this blog to stay informed, don't you? So, now you know! Of course there are many other decisions that need to be made too and these include the location of the operation and whether to go private or stay with the NHS, both of which will be determined by the type of surgery. And it looks as though there will be 5 weeks of radiotherapy to follow surgery; that is 5 weeks going to the hospital every week day! Joy!

One bit of positive news is that I had a blood test on Tuesday when I had to make an emergency trip to the eye clinic at hospital, and already my blood count was good. On the negative side, this blooming annoying eye infection will be the only reason I can't have my last chemo treatment as scheduled next Wednesday. Hopefully now that I am taking the full dose of my antibiotics (I realised yesterday that I'd got a bit confused with all the medication I've been taking and was only taking it twice a day instead of the prescribed 3 times . . . kicked myself when I realised!) this infection might finally begin to clear up.

So will I make it to the concert tomorrow? For those of you not in the know—I play the cello in the Stratford-Upon-Avon Symphony Orchestra and we have a concert tomorrow night that I've had the target of playing in for a while now. I'm making the decision in the morning—if I was a footballer they'd call it a late fitness test!

And do I have a fat enough tummy to have an option on surgery? We hope to find out on Monday. I accept that it won't *be too dreadful to have to gorge myself on cakes for the next few weeks to plump myself up a bit, but it does mean I'll have to get my trainers on that much sooner to get back in shape. On the subject of trainers and keeping in shape . . .*

I hope you don't mind, but I'd just like to introduce you to a few people at this point. There's Jo, she was in my ante-natal group; Jayne and Debbi were at University with me in Nottingham; and Clare, Tracey, Vanessa, Kate, Kim, Deanne and Sally all work with Dave for Fitness Express. If you're wondering why these ladies deserve a special mention, well, they have committed themselves to running the Race for Life this year, and have us, amongst others, in their minds as their inspiration for taking part. I've had more contact with some of these lovely ladies than I have with others over the years, but I don't think I would be doing them too much of an injustice in saying that none of them would put themselves in the 'serious runner' category (though please do correct me if I'm wrong, ladies). Jo was super-quick off the mark when it came to entering as she'll be running with no 29 on her back! I want to publicly and personally thank you all so much for donning your trainers and lycra to raise vital money to fund research into this disease, be it breast or any other type of cancer. Go girls!

I hope the sun shines for you all and I'll be on the start line with you next year (although perhaps not in Newcastle, Jayne or Swindon, Debbi!) . . .

28

Odds on Favourite

Did you get the winner on the Grand National then? I don't know about you but I'm not really the betting type and unless it's a few quid when I'm actually at the race meeting or a sweepstake in the office for the Grand National then I'm not one to bet. If I'm honest I get confused by all the odds—I mean I get the "2 to 1", "11 to 4" kind of odds but what is a "11 to 4 odds on" and is there therefore a "11 to 4 odds off"? And when you start to add in the complications of "each way" (don't they all run in the same direction?!) and spread betting—well I start to get completely lost. So it won't surprise you to know that I didn't make any money on "Ballabriggs" or any of his mates who finished close behind him on Saturday. I hope you had better luck!

Of course some of the headlines from this year's Grand National were made not by the winners but by the tragic death of two of the horses. I read a statistic that said over the past 10 years there is a 1 in 40 chance of a horse dying in that race. In other words for every 40 horses that enter only 39 come back alive. If I owned a racehorse I wonder whether that would influence my decision to enter my horse or not. The answer is I'm not sure. It's such a prestigious race and, if I owned a horse, presumably to run it in that race would be the pinnacle of achievement. But is that worth risking the horse's life? Tough call.

Those of you who caught up on Miranda's blog will know that we are reaching the next phase of her treatment and that decisions have to be made especially in relation to the type of mastectomy and subsequent breast reconstruction she has. The more advice we get the more we are given odds—there is a 1 in 200 chance that a "tummy tuck" reconstruction will fail, and the reconstructed breast tissue will die and need to be taken away. There is a 1 in 20 chance that a breast implant will be damaged by radiotherapy but there is a similar chance that, if you wait for the implant after the radiotherapy, the skin will be too tight to put the implant in as effectively. Needless to say this is a really tough decision and no conclusion has yet been reached. We have further meetings with consultants over the next few weeks to help Miranda determine the route she feels most comfortable with. We'll keep you updated I promise.

We have also got to the point where the consultants are able to give us a more accurate prognosis of the exact nature of Miranda's cancer and her long term prospects. I've learnt so much about cancer over the last four months and never appreciated the complexity of the disease. In principle, cancer is categorised into five stages from stage 0—stage 4. The higher the number the more advanced the cancer and therefore, it follows, the more difficult it is to recover from. We have now had it confirmed that Miranda's cancer is stage 3.

There is very little talk in the medical profession about being cured of cancer; they prefer to talk about 5 year and 10 year survival rates. Without doubt getting to the 5 year mark without any signs of the cancer returning is a bit of a watershed target. Having learnt a little more about Miranda's cancer there is a natural temptation to look up all the statistics on survival rates but I'm not sure how helpful that really is.

For a start, the advances over the last few years in cancer treatment have been nothing short of amazing. The drugs that make up part of Miranda's chemotherapy treatment weren't widely in use 5 years ago. So the current survival rates for breast cancer sufferers relates to people who, quite obviously, were diagnosed in 2005. Miranda is benefitting from a far more advanced treatment programme than was available then. Her survival chances must be enhanced. Furthermore although the impact of the chemotherapy on her has been significant—it has also had a massive impact on her cancer. At the last assessment, the consultant struggled to find any sense of a lump in her breast. That is so encouraging.

If you want the negative outlook then the survival rates in women under 40 years of age is lower than in older women apparently due to the fact that the cancer tends to be more aggressive in younger people. And, of course, being stage 3 means it is fairly advanced and has spread to her lymph system too. So I can tell you that there are a variety of statistics which would say that her likelihood of surviving beyond 5 years is anywhere from 40% to 70%. But my view right now is so what?

From where I stand the ultimate reality is that she will either survive to five years or she won't. What I'm interested in is not whether her chances of survival are 50%, 60%, 80% or whatever percent. I just care with a passion whether she adds to the survival or to the mortality statistics. The odds, to be honest, are irrelevant it is the outcome that matters. A bit like in the Grand National I guess, there are 39 owners who are really pleased they entered their horses and enjoyed the experience, but then there is always one owner who will forever regret the decision to have entered his horse. A 2.5%

chance of losing your horse seems small odds until it is your horse that dies.

So we will remain very positive in this household, full of determination and hope that this thing will be beaten. The final chemotherapy dose has been administered and we are about to move into the surgery stage of the battle. Miranda, as ever, is coping with the side-effects with a steely, stoical bravery. I've said it before but she is truly inspirational. To me, she really is one in a million. That's pretty long odds by the way but it's the only odds I'm really interested in for now, or for the next five years, or for the next ten years, or forever in fact.

PHASE TWO

THE MASTECTOMY

29

It's Friday—But Sunday's Coming . . . .

I don't know about you but I love the Easter story. Now I realise that many of you reading this blog won't share my Christian faith, and of course I completely respect that, but whatever your belief, or faith, I think it is difficult to deny that the actual Easter story is a good one. I mean it has pretty much everything—betrayal, greed, denial, unjust punishment, mob rule, outrageous grace, humility and ultimately hope. Hope borne out of victory against all the odds. Hope of good overcoming bad. Hope of getting through the struggles of today knowing with certainty of a better tomorrow.

It's Friday—but Sunday's coming.

I've borrowed the title of this post from one of my favourite writers, Tony Campolo, who wrote a clever book of that title that unpicks the Easter story and what it means for us today. The key thing for me in the Easter story is the hope that it brings. On Friday everything looked bleak; Jesus was dying a gruesome, brutal death on a wooden cross. If you want a flavour of how brutal it was then watch the Mel Gibson film, "The Passion of Christ"—that's about as realistic as they could make it without falling foul of the censors. All hope for Jesus' friends and followers seems lost and yet on Sunday he returns—just as he'd promised and to fulfil the predictions of the earlier prophets. Everything is restored and the world would never be the same again.

For me, the Easter story is for everyone who feels lost, let down by life, thinks their world is falling apart. It reminds us of the need to keep believing, keep trusting and know that hope is never lost.

It's Friday—but Sunday's coming.

I also love Easter as it is when the landscape changes from the barrenness of winter to the colour and new life of spring. Today has been beautiful in Suffolk and, after spending the morning in Framlingham having a coffee in the delightful "Dancing Goat" cafe and playing football with Rose and Millie at the castle, I've been in the garden cleaning the outdoor furniture, tidying up and brushing down the barbecue ready for the summer. In just a week the garden has been transformed. We are surrounded by trees many of which are in blossom and in one area we have a carpet of bluebells and forget-me-nots. We are so fortunate to live in such a setting and our garden looked so beautiful I couldn't resist taking a few photos tonight as the sun set.

So even with nature it seems that it's Friday—but Sunday's coming!

It's been Miranda's tough week, the time when the chemo is doing its worst. For those of you who have read earlier posts—this has been her "hoodie" week. Only it's been too hot for a hoodie, so for the first time she has given in and just spent the day in the house without her wig and without a hat or hoodie! It's been fine, although I think one unfortunate, delivery guy had an unnerving encounter and couldn't get away quick enough! Whilst we are on the subject of hair loss Miranda has, up until know, kept her eyelashes whilst hair everywhere else has disappeared. She was really pleased about this as she is at least able to put on some mascara and head out of the house feeling to a certain extent "made up". So it seems incredibly cruel that this last dose of chemo appears to have claimed her eyelashes with a clump coming out earlier this week. I know in the scheme of things this is fairly minor stuff but I really feel for Miranda if, at the last moment, she loses them.

We are trying to keep a perspective and humour on things of course and with her new bald look we did find ourselves having a laugh when William Hague appeared on the news in the week. Miranda and her Mum both thought he was her "looky-likey" when she is wigless!

I think this week has helped Miranda come to a decision on the type of surgery to opt for. Subject to a meeting next week with the plastic surgeon she is planning to go for the "tummy tuck" option where the breast is removed and simultaneously fat is taken from her midriff by cutting her from hip to hip(!) and reattaching it to reconstruct her breast. It's a long operation and the recovery is a bit longer too, but it is free of the need for artificial implants or pig protein and has the most realistic results apparently. The toughest part is that the operation will have to be done in Brentwood in Essex which is about 90 minutes away from us. Miranda is worried about feeling isolated. However, knowing our friends, I think there will be coach loads heading down the A12 to see her! It will present a few challenges for us as it won't be easy getting the girls to see her over the 10 days she is likely to be in hospital for, especially as Rose will be at school. But that is a short term issue and the long term outcome should be as good as we can hope for.

So the operation is likely to be in 2 or 3 weeks time. It's not far away. And when it is behind us then Miranda has to face a period of recovery and radiotherapy but then it is just the Herceptin every three weeks through to Christmas. However the side effects of that drug is minimal. Her hair will return and she won't have to write off one week in every three.

Life remains tough but you know what—it may still be Friday but Sunday's definitely coming!

Have a great Easter.

30

The Only Way is Essex

Today is the day of the Royal Wedding as Prince William marries Kate Middleton. It's the build up as I'm writing this and having told myself that I wouldn't be interested in watching it I'm finding it strangely compelling viewing! It's difficult not to get caught up in the sense of patriotism and national pride. Despite what gets written in some sections of the press it only takes an occasion like today to prove just how loved and valued the Royal Family is. There are over 150,000 people in Hyde Park alone and then there seems to be a huge number of people lining the routes between the Westminster Abbey and Buckingham Palace. Amazing and the dedication to camp out overnight! Wouldn't be for me that bit! But without a doubt as a nation we do pomp and circumstance very well don't we!

Of course there are loads of other people having their wedding today including Miranda's chemotherapy nurse Charlotte who is marrying James today at Ufford Park where we operate the health club and spa. Charlotte is having her makeup done in the spa before the event. We hope they have a wonderful and magical day just in the same way as clearly William and Kate will.

There is a lovely tenuous Ufford Park link to the Royal Wedding too! One of the page boys at the Royal Wedding is from a Suffolk family who are members of Ufford Park and he used to be looked after in our crèche while his Mum used the Club! It doesn't get more tenuous than that does it? Anyone else got an equally remote link to the Royal Wedding?!

I feel like I should post something about love and weddings but I've already done that so I'm just going to concentrate on updating you about what we have learnt this week about the next stage in Miranda's treatment programme.

We met with the consultant on Wednesday evening and the key news is that he thinks Miranda has enough body fat on her stomach to complete the "tummy tuck" procedure and so the plan is that this will happen sometime next month. He has a specialist team at the Nuffield Hospital in Brentwood and so Miranda will have to undergo the operation here. From a logistical perspective this is far from ideal being over 90 minutes away from our home. However without doubt this plastic surgeon knows his stuff so we think it is worth the upheaval. The only way really is Essex! The consultant made his name carrying out much reconstructive work on those who were amongst the worst injured in the 7/7 tube bombings. He is also amongst the 2% of consultants whose fees are so high that the healthcare insurance will only cover part of the cost and we have to make up the rest—ho hum!

I was left in complete awe at what is possible through medical advances and the skill of this surgeon. If you are slightly squeamish you may want to skip the rest of this paragraph but I think the work they are about to carry out is worthy of retelling. Miranda will have two teams working on her when they start the operation. The breast consultant will make a cut at the front of Miranda's breast and remove all the breast tissue through the hole she has created. She will also remove her lymph nodes from under her arm. Meanwhile the plastic surgeon and his team will be working on her stomach and will create a large cut through which he will painstakingly detach all the blood vessels and a chunk of fat tissue and skin. This will take him about 3 hours. They will then put the tissue back into her breast and reattach the blood vessels. Some of these vessels will be thinner than a human hair but they will all need to be stitched back together. Now there is a needle where you wouldn't want to lose the thread! The power of magnification they use to complete this work is amazing. The whole operation will take about 6 hours in total. What an incredible procedure to be able to carry out. Just amazing!

After the operation Miranda will be in the High Dependency Unit for 3 days and in hospital for a further 5/6 days before returning home. For the first few days she will have a drain on her stomach, arm and chest to remove the lymph fluid which will need to "learn" a new route through her body after the loss of her lymph nodes. Once home, she will then be able to do very little for a week before starting to recover her strength and the expectation is that she will be back to normal after 4 weeks and the scar tissue will be healed sufficiently to start radiotherapy after 6 weeks.

Aside from the obvious risks with such a big operation the biggest danger is that not all the tiny blood capillaries are reconnected in which case the reconstructed breast tissue will die and will need to be removed under emergency operation. There is about a 1 in 200 chance that this will happen but we both feel it is a risk worth taking and whatever option of reconstruction Miranda went for there would be risks and potential failures. The reconstruction should be the most realistic possible but Miranda's body doesn't recognise the change in location of the tissue. It still thinks it is stomach tissue so any fat normally stored by the body on the stomach will now be deposited on her breast. Our bodies are incredible things!

We don't have a date for the operation as Miranda still needs to meet with the anaesthetist, have a CT scan and a blood test before the consultant is happy to proceed. But we will hopefully know more after all these have been carried out over the next week. It's a busy time and although Miranda has a natural sense of trepidation about what lies ahead I think she has a much greater sense of confidence in the specialists who will be doing the work and a conviction that this is the right way to go. So we enter this next week with a sense of hope that the final tests will go OK and that we can move forward onto the next stage.

One final note is that we have received a form which once completed will allow us to enjoy a family weekend away at a venue of our choice fully paid for by a cancer trust which funds such events for cancer sufferers who are under 40. It is a lovely gesture and one more wonderful example of the great work that so many charities do to help people who are affected by this horrible disease

Today we are off for a 4 day break in North Norfolk so we'll post again from there—let's hope the sun shines although I have a nasty feeling we might be a week late!

31

A Glimpse of Heaven

Do you have a place that you can escape to? A place that, when you get there, the whole stress, worries and hassles of everyday life seem to just dissolve into the background? Well we do—and for us it is Kelling Heath Holiday Park near Holt. It is a simply beautiful holiday park offering a combination of luxurious holiday lodges, holiday homes and pitches for mobile caravans and tents, all set out within 250 acres of Norfolk countryside just a stone's throw from the sea. I don't know quite what it is that makes the place so special but from the moment we turn in the long drive I just feel a wave of tranquillity seep over me.

You know you've chosen your holiday venue well when your two children continuously shout "hooray" from the back of the car for the last five minutes of the journey as they realise where we are heading and that we have almost arrived! And that is exactly what happened as we arrived at Kelling Heath on Friday to start a 4 day break.

On the way home today Miranda and I talked about what makes Kelling Heath so special. We are well qualified to comment as we have holidayed there over 10 times in the last 5 years! We decided it was the North Norfolk location; the fact that it is privately owned and therefore not hindered by the large corporate branding and commercialism of a Center Parcs for example. That's not to say we don't like Center Parcs as we do. It is just that you get a sense with Center Parcs of it being part of a bigger organisation whereas Kelling Heath has a more personal, friendly touch. Kelling is also special due to the environmental focus of the owners which makes you feel the whole site enhances the environment rather than detracts from it; and finally the way it is laid out that makes it so peaceful. This weekend there were probably in the region of 3,500 people on the site but yet not once did it seem crowded or busy.

North Norfolk is one of my favourite parts of the country and that stretch of the coastline from Cromer around to Brancaster taking in the delights of Holkham, Morston, Burnham Market, Blakeney, Cley and Holt is just wonderful. Kelling is a few miles from Holt which is a lovely market town that gets just a little more "hip" every time we visit. Norfolk is not renowned for doing "hip" I know. Most mornings we are at Kelling we head into Holt for breakfast at Byfords—if there is anywhere that does a better breakfast I have yet to find it. It is part of our holiday tradition and they do a pretty good cappuccino too.

I can still remember the first time I went to Kelling Heath. It was about 13 years ago and we were shown around by Paul and Michael Timewell, the owners. I remember them walking us around the park and we just came to a viewing point at the top of the heath. It was as stunning then as it is now and in 13 years that vista has not changed. There is something special about looking out beyond the tiny village of Bodham and watching the sea gently amble in, the view only being interrupted by a church tower and a windmill. Every time I visit the site, whatever time of year, I always take the short walk across from the centre of the park to soak in this view. It's good for my soul.

I've been back many times as Fitness Express (the company I work for) won the contract to operate the Health

Club that the owners developed at Kelling Heath ready to open in 2000. We still operate the Club today and are working with the owners on a couple of spa projects. It is probably a bit odd to take so many holidays at a venue that is also part of my work but the only time I really feel a clash is when we go into the swimming pool. It is difficult to switch off from work mode at that point. But it must be so awful for the staff team on site too. I can't think of anything worse for them than the boss from head office pitching up to swim with his family and, as was the case this weekend, with about 20 of his mates too! They must dread being given that shift!! But, if they did, they were great as they didn't show it.

So the early May Bank sojourn to Kelling Heath has become a bit of a tradition with a group of our close friends over the last 4 years. We have had almost 50 of us there at its peak and this year there were 30 of us including the children. That's seven families in total. It is an incredibly relaxed time and we spend a lot of time sitting around talking, laughing, drinking wine and enjoying al fresco barbeque cooking. The children are impeccably behaved and it is usually the adults who are "requested" by the security to quieten down as the laughter rings around the campsite late into the evening! Despite the cold wind of this weekend we still achieved all our usual "tasks" including the customary banter with the security guard!

So now we are back home and all too soon the rest of the week looms. Rose is back to school tomorrow, I'm back to work with two London trips looming, Millie gets back to being a girl of leisure and Miranda . . . . well Miranda has a week of blood tests, a dose of Herceptin requiring a visit to the chemo club lounge, CT scan, meetings with the plastic surgeon and anaesthetist—all part of the "new normal" for her. We really hope that out of this will come a date for the mastectomy so that we can start to plan for the next few weeks and deal with this next stage of the fight.

But we do all of these things on the back of a much needed, long overdue "battery recharge" and with a sense of our spirit being uplifted. It's been a great weekend. I have no real concept of what heaven might be like but every time I drive away from a holiday at Kelling Health I feel like I've had a tiny glimpse of what it might be.

32

Its Show and Tell Time

Well I'm writing this post as the final throes of the football season are being played out with the inevitable excitement and heartbreak as the final promotion, play-off and relegation issues are resolved. As a die-hard football fan it is difficult not to get caught up in the emotion of it all and given my love of the sport it's amazing that it has taken me over 30 posts before football has got a mention in this blog! Having said that I suppose my timing could be better!

As an Ipswich Town fan it has been nothing short of a horrible season which, in reality, ended a number of weeks ago in mid-table mediocrity whilst our near neighbours and arch rivals Norwich City have capped a remarkable season with automatic promotion to the Premiership. Ouch! To make matters worse they've achieved that by playing some great football, on a shoestring budget compared to the money spent by Ipswich, and still beat us 4—1 at Carrow Road and 5—1 at Portman Road! Painful indeed!

It has been a classic lesson in the value of leadership in my opinion. Norwich City have bought in David McNally as CEO and Paul Lambert as Manager who have shown great leadership. They've made some astute purchases and assembled a group of players, none of whom are individually outstanding, but who collectively have been pretty much the best in the league. Meanwhile at Ipswich we have Simon Clegg as CEO who has allowed the best players to leave whilst failing to demonstrate any appreciation of the values of the Club and as for Roy Keane as Manager . . . . well he has struggled to transfer his incredible ability as a player into the Manager's role! Let's just say Paul Jewell, who has replaced "Keano", has a massive job on his hands! The margins between success and failure in sport are so small that it usually comes down to who has the best leadership. At Ipswich we are paying for an invisible owner and a CEO renowned for his administrative skills but who clearly lacks the ability to lead. The money that has been wasted is just shocking.

However, there is of course always someone worse off than you and poor old Grandma's team, Lincoln City, are right now about 20 minutes from dropping out of the Football League completely!

But for me, what I will remember most about this season is that I took Rose, our eldest daughter, to her first ever match. She had been keen to go for a while and I had the opportunity, thanks to a kind friend, to take her to watch a game from one of the corporate boxes last October, near her birthday. This was a perfect opportunity as I knew that if she got bored it would be easy to let her go into the box and do some drawing etc. I needn't have worried. Rose loved it! She was absorbed from start to finish and since then has learnt all the players' names. Every bedtime I now have to read through a football programme with her rather than a fairy story. Needless to say I am loving having the football, and Ipswich in particular, as a regular topic of conversation with Rose. At least I know her enthusiasm for the Tractor Boys is not borne out of a desire to follow a successful team!!

I took her to her second game in March against Scunthorpe and Ipswich won 2—0 with Jimmy Bullard scoring the second goal from a free kick. The route back to the car from the ground takes us across a large park. As we walked across the grass Rose decided to re-enact Jimmy's free kick mimicking his run up and goal celebration with remarkable accuracy. It caused much amusement for me and all those around us in the park! Needless to say I have recounted this story many times to anyone prepared to listen and I happened to mention it to a friend of mine, Simon, who is the fitness coach for Ipswich Town. He apparently relayed the story at training which led to Connor Wickham, Ipswich's 18 year old star striker, getting his shirt from that game and personally signing it for Rose! Of course the shirt has taken pride of place in Rose's bedroom—rightly so I might add!

Every Wednesday at school the children have to take something in as part of a "show and tell" activity so this week was the first chance Rose has had to take her prized shirt in. It created a bit of a stir apparently. One of the nice things about living in Suffolk is that you can be sure that the vast majority of children follow the local team. Unlike the Home Counties where the playground will certainly have a good smattering of Man Utd and Liverpool shirts; in Suffolk, Ipswich shirts always outnumber all other teams. So Rose's Connor Wickham shirt had children queuing up just to touch it! One lad even asked if he could smell it?! Rose's teacher got caught up with all the excitement too and whisked Rose off into the other class so that every child in the school saw the shirt!! Rose's school is the local village one so there are just 40 children in 2 classes! I think Rose found the attention and reaction a little overwhelming!

Miranda has been doing her own version of "show and tell" as we try to ascertain the date of her operation. A series of meetings and consultations with the various specialists involved in this stage of the treatment culminated in a CT scan yesterday. Despite this, there is still no certain date. It appears most likely that she will go into hospital next Friday (good job we are not suspicious—its Friday 13th!) and will then have her operation around 8am the following day. This is subject to the results of a final blood test on Tuesday and assumes that her infected fingernail and scratchy throat do not materialise into something more significant over the next few days.

If the mastectomy doesn't happen on 14th then Miranda will have to wait until May 30th. Although the operation and, more to the point, the recovery is not something that Miranda is particularly looking forward to I think she now just wants to get on with it. So despite a certain a sense of trepidation, she is really hoping that she gets the go ahead for next Saturday. The meetings of this week have certainly helped Miranda prepare for what lies ahead and the hospital kindly organised for her to talk to a former patient who has been through the same operation. I think this was really useful for Miranda and has helped her to be more realistic about the immediate impact of the operation coupled with the length and severity of the recovery process. Talking to this lady was like Miranda's adult version of "show and tell" really!

So I will of course keep you posted of next week's developments but for now it's time to go. The football has finished and I have a mother-in-law to console—Lincoln have been duly relegated out of the Football League. Oops!

33

Blessing in Disguise?

Isn't it strange how sometimes something that seems such a letdown or bad news can turn into a real blessing? Those of you who have followed this blog will know that we had a real disappointment about a month ago when the Breast Consultant, who has been dealing with Miranda's case, went on holiday and didn't reschedule Miranda's appointment with her and the Oncologist. It was a crucial meeting to discuss the surgery stage of the treatment that was due to follow the chemotherapy.

As Miranda described in her second guest blog post, we were pretty cross at the time. Due to the length of the consultant's holiday and the date of Miranda's last chemotherapy, we were forced to go private in order to keep the surgery within the recommended timeframe. Whilst we are covered for this, it felt at the time like a bit of an unnecessary distraction with the added hassle of claims forms and we had, up to that point, been so happy with the quality, efficiency and friendliness of the care Miranda had received under the NHS.

However by going private Miranda has been brought under the care of a Breast Consultant, Ms Aitken, who is known to the team at the NHS hospital in Ipswich as she worked there until recently and who, more importantly, Miranda feels a really great affinity with. Furthermore, Ms Aitken works with a plastic surgeon who will carry out the reconstruction and who seems to be amongst the best in his field. I "googled" him and found an article in a Sunday newspaper from a few months ago which had him listed in the top ten consultants in the UK who leading medics would use if they need plastic surgery. He does have an air of calming reassurance and confidence about him which both Miranda and I find very comforting. We know that this mastectomy and reconstruction is a significant operation. It will last for 6/7 hours and Miranda will be in the High Dependency Unit for 48 hours afterwards. But I genuinely don't think that Miranda could have a better team working on her. And we have only got this team because someone at the NHS was incapable of scheduling an appointment.

Annoying at the time but it's turned out to be a real blessing in disguise.

Without doubt Miranda has found this part of the programme the toughest yet and I think that's possibly because she has had options. Up until now the decisions about her treatment have been out of her hands. The chemo has been horrible but it has also been inevitable and completely in the control of the consultants. With the mastectomy an element of choice has been introduced and Miranda has needed to take on board the comments of the specialists and then make her own decision as to the best way forward. When we first discussed the options she faced she would look at me and say words to the effect of:

"I don't want any of them really!"

However, rather in the style of Ted Rogers and his "3-2-1" programme with "Dusty Bin" (for those of you who go back as far as me and can remember the delights of 1980's Saturday night TV), we have gradually rejected treatment options and have genuine confidence that the final remaining option—the "tummy tuck"—is the right procedure for Miranda.

By the way I can still do that 3-2-1 thing by spinning my fingers just like old Ted used to do—can you?

Thanks to the support, advice and reassurance of the medical team now working with her, Miranda has a sense of peace about the decision she has made coupled with a determination to get on and deal with it and put the whole process behind her. The wait for this Friday and her admittance to hospital has been hard for all of us though. Rose has shed a few tears on a number of occasions at the thought of her Mum being in hospital for 10 days, I'm feeling a high degree of tension about the whole process, and I think Miranda just wants to get the inevitable trauma done and put behind her. So the last few days have been a bit stressful.

You can imagine therefore our complete frustration and disappointment when her latest blood test results came back yesterday and her white cell count was too low for the operation to proceed as planned this weekend! It is now scheduled for June 4th. That seems a long way away. It is way beyond the timeframe that the oncologist had initially set for the mastectomy to happen, although Miranda has been reassured that this is not a major concern. It is better to wait for her white cell count to increase so that her body is able to heal quicker and more effectively. The delay in the operation will obviously push back her radiotherapy. This has the knock on effect of meaning our family summer holiday will now have to be cancelled and worst of all, apparently(?!), Miranda is going to miss a Take That concert! All pretty rubbish really (I'm talking here about all the upheaval not the Take That concert obviously!!)

However in typical, indomitable Miranda spirit she has bounced back from this new disappointment and last night announced that the delay is for the best. To have rushed the operation through this weekend could have meant her body wouldn't have been able to effectively fight any infection that got into her wounds, potentially making her even more ill. She's decided that she has now gained 3 more weeks of feeling well and able to enjoy life. More time can be spent getting on top of the vegetable garden, potting out our tubs and hanging baskets, and organising the netting for the fruit cage.

Miranda has also decided that before the op the two of us will have a night away in Holt, our favourite North Norfolk bolthole, and we now get to go to the Safari Supper in the village, which is always a cracking night out. Our family holiday is being rescheduled for the last week of the school holidays and we will go away to our original destination in the autumn half term too, hopefully.

So maybe the delay will turn out to be another blessing in disguise. It's just that yesterday morning it felt very well disguised!

After a tearful conversation with her in the morning when the news came through, I got home last night wondering what state everyone would be in and fearing there may be tension in the air. I walked in the back door and found Miranda, Rose and Millie in the kitchen all doing the "hokey cokey"! I dropped my work bag, Miranda cued the CD back to the start and the four of us laughed our way through the whole routine. It's a well established fact in our household that laughter is by far the best medicine.

I know I'm biased but I do think Miranda is an amazing girl with just an incredible spirit and determination!

Well that's more than enough from me for tonight but before I go could you just do this with me for a moment. Could you . . . . put your left arm in . . . . your left arm out . . . . in . . . out . . . in . . . out . . . . and shake it all about you do the hokey cokey and you turn around . . . . that's what it's all about!!

Indeed it is!

34

That's What Friends Are For

Last week Harriet, Rose's school friend, left the school and moved out of the area. It's a real shame for Rose and from her point of view the timing was pretty awful coming as it does when she is struggling a little with the thought of her Mum's impending hospital stay. Rose told us that she was really sad and as we weren't aware of Harriet's departure we hadn't had the chance to prepare her for it. As I've mentioned before Rose's school is tiny—it comprises just 40 pupils split into 2 classes across the 7 years. There were only 5 girls in Rose's year group and now there are 3 left. That is not a good number. On Monday Rose admitted that she had spent most of playtime by herself and said "Mummy—I'm going to have to think of a really good show and tell as that will get me some friends."

It was a comment that we found a little bit amusing and an awful lot heartbreaking to be honest. Clearly the "Show and Tell" which Rose did with her personally signed Connor Wickham shirt a few weeks ago has left a big impression with her. It meant she became the centre of attention for a while and everyone wanted to talk to her.

It gave us an opportunity to explain to Rose what real friendship means. To explain that the best way to get friends is to be one. That we need to understand that some people will be friendly because we have something they want or are interested in (like a Connor Wickham shirt!) but that true friends are the kind of people who are interested in us for who we are, who will stick by us when the going gets tough and who we really enjoy spending time with too.

I really hope it is a lesson that she will learn, remember and apply over the coming years.

It also reminded us how fortunate we are to have wonderful friends who support us in so many ways. At times it has been a little overwhelming. Only today I rang a business associate to talk about an idea I had that I thought might solve a business problem we are both challenged by. Before I had chance to explain why I was calling he was asking after Miranda and offering words of support and encouragement that were far more helpful and appreciated than he could probably ever realise. I've had two emails from one of my best buddies just checking that I was OK whilst my best friend of almost 40 years has shown incredible understanding over us changing arrangements for his visit this weekend. And a card arrived from some friends in Birmingham just letting us know that we are in their thoughts. That's just today!

It's all been really timely as, if truth be told, the last few days have been tougher for Miranda than she was expecting. She has been a little emotional and the reality of what lies ahead is weighing heavy on her mind. Perfectly understandable but still pretty horrible. I think there are a number of reasons why she feels like this. Clearly, whilst offering some advantages, the long wait for her surgery is not helping. It's a massive operation but the thought of it can often be worse than the reality and Miranda is getting a lot of thinking time. She is also still feeling the side-effects of the final chemo, probably more than she expected to. Her latest problems are achy legs, hot flushes and tiredness. Today's blood test identified that her red blood cells and platelets are normal but her white blood cell count and "neutrophils" (don't ask me what these are—it's just something to do with white blood cells and fighting infection!) are really low. This isn't a major issue as there is still time before the operation but she will be tested again next week when she goes for her next dose of Herceptin.

So it's been a difficult few days. Miranda has been telling me how she doesn't feel very brave anymore and how she's a little more fearful about the future.

The antidote to this has been for Miranda to meet with some friends last night, to cry with a little and pray with a lot. She has a few lunches set up and today there was a bit of retail therapy too.

She will come through this of course. I know she will—I keep reminding myself that this is Miranda we are talking about after all! But in the meantime we are leaning on a number of people who are around us. We are so grateful for them.

And when all this is over, when this disease is beaten, when this blog is finished and forgotten, when this journey is over, maybe we will have the chance to provide the same support to them at some point.

After all that's what friends are for isn't it?

35

Going on Safari

So since we last got together on the blog Miranda and I have been on a safari! I promise we really have! But before I tell you all about it let me just explain this to you . . .

I'm writing this blog on the way back from a work trip to Manchester. Opposite me is sitting a guy who obviously works for a food distributor. Right now he is on the phone getting animated about the "broccoli problem" and on his last call he demanded to know if his office had sorted the "cauliflower issue". He is keeping me amused and I'm really fighting the temptation to ask him if he could expand on the broccoli problem for me! The only broccoli problem we have is when Rose refuses to eat hers because it is too soft. At 5 she is already a bit of a food critic you see.

It's just made me realise how much we get wrapped up in our own little world and what becomes part of everyday life for us sounds really odd to others. It would be great wouldn't it, if my travelling companion was writing his blog about this strange guy opposite him who just had a conversation about putting together an offer on pedicures and self tanning as that's what I have just done with one of our Spa Managers!

On the way up this morning I was sat with two old boys who were out on a day of train spotting. They were off to Nuneaton as apparently "there's an awful lot of freight that goes through there". They were hoping to spot a new type of freight locomotive which may be heading that way.

When they weren't engrossed in talk about trains they were swapping photos of buses and trams which they also clearly took an interest in—clearly broad minded train spotters these guys! All the way through the journey I just wanted to ask them; why? I mean where is the pleasure in traipsing across the country to see a few passing locomotives so you can scribble the engine number down in a little book! Really? And even if they do want to do that then could they at least explain—Nuneaton?! Honestly! At least choose a nice station with a Starbucks on it!!

But that's the thing—we are all so different. They probably would not understand why I still feel a bit sore about the fact that my beloved Ipswich Town got tonked 5—1 at home by Norwich. But I am—it is still a painful memory for me! The fact that we are so different is what makes me so fascinated by people. I could sit and people watch all day if given the chance. The fact we are all so different is what makes the art of delivering great customer service just that—an art not a science. What is great service for one individual is either over attentive or just not what's expected by another. And that is the challenge and the fun of my job and why I love it so much. I'm so grateful to all the teams I work with who everyday try to fathom out how to tailor what we do to exceed every one of our members and guests expectations. It's a real challenge but it is great fun too.

In any situation, even on a train, I love finding out what makes people tick and what their world is about. So you will understand why I loved our Saturday night safari. It was a kind of people and food safari. We live in a beautiful, small Suffolk village with less than 400 inhabitants and last weekend was the annual village safari supper. The theme is that everyone gets allocated a house to turn up at for a starter course. Each host house entertains around 8 people and from there everyone is sent off to different houses for their main course before we all end up at the same, rather large house for desserts.

There were 14 host houses and over 60 people who "safari'd" that night. Normally Miranda hosts but this year we weren't expecting to be able to go, never mind host. So it was an added bonus and, as ever, a cracking night. We've been going for three years now and each time we meet people who we've never met before but who live in our village. It is such a cool idea and I'm in my element. This year I met a lady who restores ancient paintings, a guy who works at the Sizewell nuclear plant and whose wife helps build self-esteem and confidence in people with depression whilst at our "main course" house I met a guy who is an accountant for a company whose turnover makes what my business does look like loose change.

Everyone had a great story to tell and I loved hearing a little about them, as well as catching up with some of the friends we have met previous years or who we just know so well. At the "starter house" I even got chance to reminisce with my mate Jim who I played cricket with for a number of years. Isn't it funny how you always remember the games you won! We talked about the year we won the Suffolk Federation Cup and then remembered that we must be getting old if we are talking about the past!

It was a lovely evening and a chance to forget about Miranda's illness for a while. Not everyone knew she had cancer and those that did chose not to talk about it which for that one night was really lovely. It was like we had escaped back for a while into what life was like before her diagnosis and we both felt better for that kind of night out. I even drove, so Miranda could enjoy some well earned Pimms followed by wine through the evening! Good times.

Meanwhile back to reality and the wait goes on for Miranda's mastectomy. She has her next dose of Herceptin tomorrow (Wednesday) and will have more blood tests tomorrow. The date of June 4th seems pretty definite and there is talk of artificially boosting her blood count prior to then if it hasn't increased naturally.

The excitement for me this week centres on a planned return flight to Edinburgh on Friday as the news breaks of major airline disruption due to the Icelandic volcano. I haven't got a good record with ash clouds, having been stuck in Split for a week with the last eruption. Still that led to my first attempt at blogging—"Time to Split"—so it could make a good story to retell.

And that is the point really—we do all have a story to tell and I loved hearing other peoples on Saturday as we went on "safari". We are all on a journey—and each of us will experience some exciting points and some not so exciting. This quote from the poet and novelist, Nancy Willard, found its way into my email inbox today and I thought it was worthy of sharing with you:

> *"I haven't a clue how my story will end, but that's all right. When you set out on a journey and night covers the road, that's when you discover the stars."*

Miranda and I are learning to accept the uncertainty of travel plans and accept that what defines us is not so much the journey, but the way we travel. Just so happens that for a while we travel in darkness and therefore will get the opportunity to discover a few stars. And I suppose that's no bad thing really . . . .

36

The Tapping Finger

Well the good news is that this week Miranda's blood tests came back showing that her count was up. What a relief! There was a glimmer of concern last week from her Oncologist that the low readings might indicate that Miranda's bone marrow was being a little slow to recover from the onslaught of chemotherapy but this week's results have ended that worry. The levels are such that if all remains the same then her operation will proceed exactly a week today. Miranda will be so very glad to put that behind her. However, without wishing to be alarmist, she is feeling pretty rough today with a sore throat and a cold. We have everything crossed that this doesn't develop into something that means she is either too unwell or causes her blood count to drop thus preventing the op happening.

It feels like we have been living life on tenterhooks for a while now. A couple of weeks ago Miranda found herself reading a newspaper article about a guy who had got breast cancer. There seems to be a bit of focus on men and breast cancer in the media at the moment although the incidence of this type of the disease is still relatively rare in men. According to the latest stats from Cancer Research around 300 men a year are diagnosed with breast cancer, which equates to 1 man for every 150 women who contract the disease. The problem was that the symptoms for this guy were remarkably similar to Miranda's and after his chemo, and being given the all clear, the cancer sadly spread sometime later to other organs and he ultimately lost his battle for life. Obviously for Miranda, who has been experiencing a bit of neck pain lately (no jokes about me being a pain in the neck for her please!), this was not easy reading. Coupled with a few other unexplained aches and pains and the fact she still feels pretty rough from the chemo, it has left her understandably feeling anxious and worried.

She called Rachel, her "key support" nurse and who has been wonderfully supportive over the past few months and got much of the reassurance that she needed. Rachel is always encouraging but always realistic and explained that Miranda is likely to still feel the effects of the chemo for up to a year. At least we now know that. What Rachel also said was that it was perfectly natural to have the doubts and fears that Miranda has had over the past few weeks.

"You'll go for ages without thinking anything about it but then you will see, hear or read something and that finger of doubt will be tapping on your shoulder. You need to accept that this tapping finger will never completely go away" she explained

I remember when Miranda was first diagnosed Rachel telling us that so many cancer victims found the period after treatment was the toughest part of the illness. They recover from the operation, the chemo, and the radiotherapy but they can't recover from the doubt of the cancer coming back. At the time that just seemed so incongruous but I now realise what she means. The fear of the unknown is somehow much harder to deal with than the reality of the situation you face, irrespective of how tough that situation might be.

But Rachel has got me thinking to be honest. I think that we all have a tapping finger on our shoulder don't we? It might be a sense of self doubt, worries about work, our relationships, whatever it is we all have to learn to deal with that regular tap on the shoulder. Sometimes I have to make fairly bold and significant decisions at work. For those of you who are involved in that part of my life and see the confidence with which I announce and implement them please don't let that kid you that there isn't a tapping finger on my shoulder about whether I've done the right thing or not.

But what I've come to realise is that looking back, I regret far more the times when I listened and responded to the tapping finger of doubt than I regret the times when I ignored it and took the bold decision. So I think that Rachel's advice to Miranda has helped remind me that life is not about the tapping finger or what it "taps us" about—it's about how we respond. Do we turn round and take notice every time or do we just ignore it and carry on anyway? And as I'm putting this post together I'm also fully aware that it's easy to write about what we should do and not so easy to put into practice. I'd hate to give you the impression that Miranda or I have any great insight or wisdom into how to ignore that "tap" on the shoulder. Indeed it feels a pretty big distraction right now to be honest.

But what I do know is this.

Whether we let that tapping finger interfere with our lives and what we do with it or not, the ultimate outcome will still be the same. I remember a powerful talk at the Forge about how if you look at someone's gravestone there is a start date for when they were born and an end date when they died and between the two dates there's a small dash. Now we have absolutely no influence over the start date and no real impact on when the end date is.

However the bit in the middle, the dash, is completely down to us. So the key part of the message was what are we doing with our dash?

For Miranda and I that tapping finger is trying to make us think about the end date arriving for her way, way sooner than we ever imagined or would want. Maybe it will, maybe it won't. Who knows? We can't really do much about it. So no matter how loud the tap we are trying with all our effort to ignore it. Drown it out in fact with the fun and laughter of our dash. And if you had been in Rose's ballet class this morning and seen me try to take part I promise you would have found plenty of chances to laugh! A lot more awkward stumble than dash to be fair!

Obviously the last few months have been full of more doubt and worry for us than at any other time in both our lives. Going through Miranda's battle with cancer with her has made me focus on my life and what I'm doing with it more than ever before. And it's the same for Miranda too. And how about you? Is there a tapping finger on your shoulder that's infecting what you do too much? If there is, I hope in some tiny way our story may help you to ignore it and just focus on how you are filling your dash. It's just a thought. Anyway that's more than enough from me I need to get on.

Must dash in fact . . . .

37

Somewhere Over the Rainbow

You know that when the secretary of your wife's Consultant rings and asks her to come in and see the Consultant that afternoon; and that when you get there and explain that you will take the children off to the play area in the waiting room and the Consultant says "No I think you had better come in as well" that she has probably not good news for you. And that's exactly how it was today.

The news is that Miranda's white blood cell count which, as mentioned in the previous post, has been slow to recover from the chemotherapy is actually of greater concern than we had previously been led to believe. Seven weeks after chemo finished and, although steadily increasing, it is well below normal and this is pretty unusual at this stage. Less than 1 in 10 people have this reaction. It means that the Oncologist, Breast Consultant and Plastic Surgeon have collectively decided that it is too low for them to safely carry out the mastectomy and breast reconstruction. To do so would mean Miranda is open to a significant risk that her body would be unable to fight any potential infection resulting from the wounds the operation would leave her with. That scenario could be potentially life-threatening. They also feel that we have run out of time to wait any longer because of the increasing delay between the chemo and the radiotherapy treatments.

So the new plan is that she will have two more blood tests, tomorrow and next week, and a simple mastectomy on June 13th assuming the white blood cell count increases to a safe level. Once she has recovered from the surgery then radiotherapy will start and any reconstruction will have to wait until September of next year. That seems a very long way away.

Of course part of the conversation today centred around the plan if the white blood cells don't increase. The reality is that they will need to investigate why the bone marrow is not returning to normal and this could include taking a sample of bone marrow to test—not a particularly pleasant procedure. The expected cause is that it is simply the effect of the chemotherapy, but there is also a small chance that the cancer could now have spread to Miranda's bone marrow and they want to rule that possibility out. Given the profile of her other blood counts this is very unlikely and is not something we want to even contemplate right now. But if the count doesn't increase then it would appear the specialists have to weigh up the risk of an operation and possible infection, with the risk of delaying the radiotherapy treatment and thereby increasing the chance of the cancer returning to the affected areas. I'm glad that is a call that I don't have to make. But I wish with all my heart that they don't have to make that call about my wife either. The tension of waiting for those blood tests is feeling a bit of a challenge too right now.

So, all in all, today's news has been a bit of a hammer blow to be honest. It has been hard news to take for both of us, but especially Miranda, who now has to get her head around the fact that she is not going to have immediate breast reconstruction. The desire to wake up from her mastectomy with a reconstructed breast was the one thing that she was certain about with this stage of the treatment.

So please forgive us for taking the easy route of updating you all through this blog with the news as the thought of telling everyone individually feels a bit daunting at the moment.

And I've reread my "Blessing in Disguise" post and am trying to convince myself that today's news falls into that category. Maybe it does but I can't see it right now. However, as with any situation there are always some positives, Miranda will now have the operation in Ipswich, will be in hospital for less time, will recover quicker and oh yes—we have the most amazing children—within 15 minutes of being back in the house Rose had drawn and written a "hope you are feeling better soon Mummy" card. So perceptive for a 5 year old.

But it all seems small comfort against the backdrop of today's meeting. Inevitably, and almost for the first time since we discovered this horrible disease had come into Miranda's life, we found ourselves asking the "why" questions. Why is this happening? Why does the situation seem to just get worse and not better? Why is Miranda going to have to deal with the psychological and physical challenges of the mastectomy? Why? Why?

So we got a bit angry, we cried a bit and I read Miranda the closing paragraphs of Rob Bell's book "Love Wins" to try to get us more positive. It's a brilliant, incisive book, as all Rob Bell's books tend to be, and it's main message is that through everything we experience and all that we do God loves us and that love will win through;

> *"May you experience this vast, expansive, infinite, indestructible love that has been yours all along.*

147

> *May you discover that this love is as wide as the sky and as small as the cracks in your heart no one else knows about.*
>
> *And may you know deep in your bones, that love wins"*

That is how the book closes and we found it moving but challenging in that moment. Shortly afterwards the most amazingly beautiful rainbow appeared in the sky above our house.

A symbol of hope when we most needed it.

Somehow we need to find a way across it to the other side and leave behind the challenges we currently face—I'm not sure how we do this right now but we will get there. Stick with us won't you.

38

Everyone's Normal
Until You Get to Know Them

I realise that I'm in danger of this blog seeming as though it is sponsored by John Ortberg! I've borrowed the title of this post from one of his older books having quoted passages of another book previously. But the thing is, it is so true—everyone does seem so normal until you get to know them really well, and then you realise all their quirks, foibles and jagged edges. Just ask Miranda sometime, and she happily let you know about all the things that make me further from normal than you could ever imagine!

And the odd thing is that "normal" gets a bit of a bad press really doesn't it? I mean to be "normal" is almost a bit derogatory. "Normal" can sometimes be a bit boring, a bit grey.

Legend has it that there is an official medical condition in East Anglia which is known as "normal for Norfolk" and although I can't believe that's true I couldn't resist mentioning it! After all there is not much opportunity for those of us south of the East Anglian border to put one over on our Norfolk rivals after Norwich's promotion to the Premiership!

However in our household we crave a bit of normality right now to be honest, such has been the challenge of the past few months. So today we are thrilled to learn that

Miranda, or at least her white blood cell count, is normal. It is so lovely to be normal! Her count from the test of today is up to 5.6 having been 4.8 last week and 3.3 the week before. Wonderful, wonderful news!

It means that, saving a complete curveball thrown in from the consultant at tomorrow's meeting, Miranda's operation will go ahead on Monday. I almost feel I need to add in our mantra of "expect the unexpected" here. She has to "check-in" to the hospital at 7am and in a strange kind of way we are almost looking forward to it happening—it's something that is inevitable and unavoidable so we want to put it behind us.

Thank you so much for the amazing reaction to last week's news regarding the blood test and the impact on the type of operation Miranda can now have. The comments on the blog, facebook, twitter and via text were both wonderful and overwhelming. I'm sorry if I didn't get time to reply to all of them but we really did appreciate your support.

Assuming there is no more dramatic late changes to the plan then I will put a blog up on Monday morning so that you can all be certain that the operation is going ahead. I will also post up as a comment on that same post Monday evening to let you know how everything has gone.

I think it is impossible to calculate how Miranda will feel afterwards, especially as there can be no reconstruction for over a year, but like everything else she has faced so far, I'm sure she will find a way of dealing with it. Let's face it she is pretty amazing, incredibly strong and determined. An inspiration to me and the girls that's for sure.

Indeed she has even asked me to point out to you that every cloud has a silver lining and that the simpler operation means that she can reclaim her Take That ticket. She now has a certain concert in early July to look forward to. Now that is certainly not normal is it?!

Not normal at all. But then again, everyone's normal until you get to know them aren't they?

39

Riding the Zip Wire

It's finally here then. In fact it is happening right now. As I sit here in Starbucks sipping anxiously on my tall, skinny cappuccino Miranda is a few miles away undergoing a mastectomy.

If all goes to plan it will take the surgeon just over an hour to carry out the main procedure in addition to removing all of the lymph nodes that are under her arm for good measure. A temporary drain will be fitted to help her lymphatic system work out a new "route" around her body and then it will all be over. Back to the recovery room and, after a further hour or so coming round, I will be able to see her.

All sounds so simple but yet it is a process that will have significant physical and potential psychological impact. The loss of the lymph nodes, will consign Miranda to a lifetime of susceptibility to lymphedema, a condition which causes the swelling of the arm and for which there is no surgical cure just treatment with physio and compression bandages.

All sounds a bit brutal . . . . but then it is actually.

Since dropping her off at 7am this morning and waiting around for the pre-op formalities to be complete, I've driven into Ipswich, fretted a lot, prayed a bit and it probably should have been the other way around. And now I've ended up in Starbucks doing what I have always done when I'm struggling with this evil disease that's become part of everyday life for my family—I'm writing to you to tell you what I'm thinking.

On the drive across from the hospital I've been trying in my mind to find the words to adequately convey how it feels right now. And it's been really difficult to find them to be honest. Indeed the best way that I've come up with is to tell you a story . . . .

It goes back about three years, around the time that Millie was born, when I took Rose to the park at Framlingham to give Miranda a bit of a break. It's a lovely park with lots of different play equipment including a zip wire. Rose always enjoyed the zip wire even though she was a bit young for it at the time. I'd been gently sending her down a few times and we were just about to leave. "One more time Daddy" was the request, and then "it" happened. I am sure that if I was cleverer there is some amazing scientific formula that could explain "it" but I'm not, so I have no idea why. But you see, without any extra perceived effort on my part I sent Rose down on the zip wire one last time. This time, however, the moment I let go of the pole she just flew down the wire at breakneck speed.

To this day I cannot explain why, maybe the angle of release of my arm was in perfect symmetry with the angle of the pole, or the increasing heat from previous go's removed all friction from the wire, or if you believe in the chaos theory of nature, maybe a butterfly broke wind in Borneo and the resultant ripple effect created a thermal current just at the wrong moment in Fram park. But whatever it was I knew from the moment I let go that I had no chance of catching Rose before she got to the end of the wire. All I could do was stand there and wait and hope that she managed to hold on to the pole. It was one of those occasions when it felt like time froze.

I watched as the runners on the wire reached the stopper at the end and then the pole, to which Rose clung, just kept on going; swinging up in a dramatic arc like some out of control pole vault. There was a point when Rose was almost horizontal with the wire and the ground. I calculated in my head that if she let go at the top of the arc she would clear the silly springy toy with the wooden painted hedgehog on it, the bench where sensible parents sit and watch their children playing, and the fence that borders the park; projecting herself into the back garden of a neighbouring bungalow. Now many was the time as a boy when I kicked a football out of the park and into someone's back garden and I remember the embarrassment of having to go and ask for it back. In my mind I spooled forward to the type of conversation I might have if the same fate happened to Rose.

I imagined knocking on the door of some old lady and saying something like—"I'm really sorry but I was playing with my daughter in the park and, completely by accident, she has inadvertently landed up in your back garden. Could I have her back please?"

And the reply would be something like "Yes dear—I'll get her just this once but if it happens again then I might not be so happy" and then as she heads off to her back door adding something like "I may be a moment or two getting her as I don't know the number for social services off the top of my head"!

Anyway Rose clung on and as she came back down I was there to grab her and the pole. She didn't cry. Neither of us spoke. We hugged and then gave each other a little look to confirm that we had both found it as scary as the other and we walked back to the car in silence. After a while I suggested it was best we probably didn't tell her Mum what happened and Rose agreed that she thought that was a really good idea. Of course she's never let me push her on a zip wire ever again.

I can laugh about it now but at the time . . . .

Now I tell that story, partly for the inevitable smile it brings to my face, and hopefully yours too, but also because that moment when I let go of Rose and watched her hurtle away from me, not knowing what would happen when she got to the end of the wire. That moment when I let go and could do nothing but wait and hope and stand helpless, watching her desperately cling to the pole. That emotion of utter disbelief and helplessness that I had then. That is the best way of explaining how I feel right now.

I know I've had six months to get my head around it but I still have plenty of occasions when I cannot believe that Miranda has cancer. It is as surreal now as it was when we first found out. I picked up a leaflet at the hospital the other day and read of the eight most common risk factors associated with breast cancer, Miranda had only one of them—she is a woman. All the other risk factors don't apply to her. How can that be? How did it end up in her body when there is so little evidence to suggest that she is susceptible? The disbelief of her cancer is as strong as ever this morning.

And the helplessness kills me. I am a bloke (no prizes if you'd already guessed this by the way!) and so I need to do practical things or find solutions. I don't do empathy and understanding without action very well. The standing on the sidelines watching, whilst Miranda battles through everything that has been thrown at her over the last six months, has been so painful and today is perhaps the toughest yet. I simply don't have the ability to describe how I felt as I just stood and watched the nurses wheel my incredibly brave and beautiful wife down the corridor to the operating theatre. Through the inevitable tears she was still managing a smile. And now, well, I mean I'm just sat here drinking coffee whilst she is . . . . you can imagine how useless I feel can't you?

But before I start to wallow in a sea of self-pity the other thoughts which keep pushing their way to the forefront of my mind is how much I have to be grateful for. This blog is all about my story and the journey I'm on with my wife and daughters but there are others who are travelling on a much tougher road. I could tell the story of our friend Laura whose 3 year old son has a serious heart and lung condition that the doctors have never seen before. Then there is Dan and Jen who with their 3 young boys have "upped sticks" and gone to South Africa to help bring practical help to orphans who lack the basics of clean water, health care and education. The stories Dan tells about the children he encounters everyday make me realise how truly blessed I, and Rose and Millie, really are. The journey they are on, makes mine look like a relative walk in the park.

And finally there is the God thing going around my head too this morning. In telling our story I've tried really hard to share a bit about our Christian faith and what we believe in without sounding pious, judgemental or too pushy. I recognise that there are many of you reading this who share that faith and many who don't, and wherever you sit on this issue we so appreciate you following our story and the support that gives us. I so want everyone to feel valued by us, irrespective of your faith or belief structure.

Over the past few months a number of people have asked me questions about my faith and how I reconcile it with what is going on right now. The most common questions seem to be around "has my faith been tested by this" and "how can I possibly think there is a loving God when Miranda has to suffer in the way she does". They are both really valid questions and each is worthy of a blog in its own right and maybe one day I will have a go at writing them.

But not this morning.

Right now I just feel compelled to say that I can completely understand how people who go through what Miranda and I are experiencing turn away from God and find their faith diminished. I will confess to, at times, feeling an element of anger and a little bit of bitterness. And when you are in that position it is easy to put God in the firing line.

But what I know, without doubt, is that God never promises us an easy life or a life that is free from hurt, pain or challenges. A Christian faith is not an insurance policy that protects us from the difficulties and suffering that everyday life can throw at us. Rather, what God does promise, is that He will be with us always and that He will be closest to us when the going gets tough. And, best of all, He provides the hope of a better future, both in this life and beyond. To walk with that hope in our hearts enables anyone to cope with the toughest of challenges and, for me, provides the greatest sense of affirmation about my faith.

So right now, as I sit here finishing my second coffee and preparing to return to the hospital to find out how my wife has come through this latest horrible experience, I feel that I need to be thankful to God and for the hope that He brings. I need to be thankful to Him for being so close to me right now that I can almost sense His breath on my cheeks—in Starbucks of all places too! And I feel that I need to tell you of that fact too.

And I know, above all else that is happening to us right now, I need to cling on to Him, and the hope that He brings, with the same sense of white-knuckled desperation that Rose clung to that pole on the zip wire three years ago.

2:30pm Blog Update

All is well and Miranda is back from the theatre. I've been with her for about 30mins. She is very sleepy which is only to be expected! The operation was successful and although Miranda can't really remember what the consultant said it appears that there was no sign of any remaining cancer in either her breast or the lymph nodes which is fantastic although I am looking forward to hearing that first hand rather than from a woozy wife! Of course Miranda being Miranda is refusing all morphine at the moment whilst I on the other hand am slightly tempted!! Only slight concern is the numbness in her arm which is hopefully due to some anaesthetic rather than a damaged nerve. Consultant due around 6pm so will update again after that. Thanks for all the prayers and good wishes—they worked it seems!

5:30pm Blog Update

So the consultant has been around and I have the official update! It is true that all the indications are that the cancer has gone but they are only visual checks. The real key test is when the tissues that have been removed are analysed under the microscope. So it's good but we're not getting carried away too soon.

Miranda is much more awake now and, having had her first wee (always a key post op moment!) is now tucking into her supper. Her humour has returned even telling the consultant when she walked back in the room that she reminded her of the Paul Young song "Every Time You Go Away, You Take a Piece of Me With You"!! It's amazing how black humour soon enters the dialogue. Even I told Miranda

I needed to update the blog to keep everyone abreast of the situation!

So I'm about to head home and see the girls before their bedtime. So relieved to see Miranda in such good spirits! She is still a little light headed—probably not helped by me having the remote control for the bed upside down so sending her back horizontal when she was expecting to be lifted up to drink her tea. I'm a class act!

Thanks again for all your support and encouragement throughout the day. Miranda has loved hearing your comments although she may not quite remember them all! Goodnight!

40

Mummy's on the Mend

Hello everyone—it's Rose here. I hope you don't mind but me and my sister Millie have found out how to get onto Daddy's blog and we thought it was time that we had chance to tell you how we are doing. My sister is very clever on the computer even though she is not quite 3—she can find most children's TV programme websites within a few clicks. She has got us onto the blog and I am putting the words together—this spellchecker thing is very clever isn't it? Without that you might not work out every word as although I can talk fine my spellings not the best—but then again I am only 5!

Daddy is complaining of being really tired—he says it might be all the worry or something. Goodness knows why he should be tired—I mean me and Grandma are having to do all the organising, making sure he is doing the right things in the right order and generally looking after him. If anyone is going to be tired it should be me and Grandma. As the oldest lady in the household I realise it is my job to take charge. I know Grandma is an awfully lot older than me but she doesn't count as she is only really a guest here and has her own house. I know Mummy has done blogs before and so I thought I should step in while she isn't around. And let's face it Daddy does go on a bit doesn't he! His last blog was over 2,000 words long—I was very bored by the time he'd finished reading it to me I can tell you.

So let me tell you about Mummy. She is doing very, very well. Her op went well and the consultant is very pleased with her. She generally feels OK. I don't really understand all what is going on but Daddy said the consultant told him that what she found was as good as we could have hoped for. Daddy told me that Mummy might be a bit upset after the op but of course she wasn't when I saw her—she was as smiley as ever. I know my Mummy and I knew she would be fine about things. She gets a bit tired especially when her friends Tracey and Lisa go to see her as they make her laugh loads and mess about.

Me and Millie went to see Mummy on Tuesday and I was surprised to see how well she looked. She had a new pair of pyjamas on and she had put her wig on. This is a good sign—when Mummy's poorly she doesn't wear her wig. Her hair is really growing back now and Daddy says she is timing it to perfection as her head looks like a tennis ball just in time for Wimbledon! He is a bit silly sometimes. He has been itching to tell everyone that it is growing back with a bit more grey in it but he knows Mummy would be really cross if he put that in a blog. She never gets cross with me so I'm sure she won't mind that I've told you—you'll find out before too long anyway.

She still has a "thing" in her with a long tube that is collecting some blood type stuff and she has to carry a shopping bag around with her all the time with a collection bottle in it. Mummy hopes to come home on Friday and she thinks she may not have to bring the bottle or the tubes. That would be really good. Mummy's room at the hospital is lovely. By the way my sister can't say hospital she calls it "hopeeetal". Daddy says that is where poorly bunny rabbits should go. We try not to laugh too much as it only encourages him.

After we had been with Mummy for a while we went out of her room onto the garden. She has her own patio doors and there was a big garden for me to run in. It is very lovely and leads down to the woods. I've just been reading a book about going on a bear hunt. So me, Millie and Daddy pretended we were going on a bear hunt and ran around for ages. When I was going back to find Mummy I couldn't remember which was her patio doors and then amazingly I heard this man calling out "bear" really loudly a few times from his bed through the open patio doors. I thought this was amazing that he had actually found a bear when we had just pretended we were hunting one. Daddy was with Millie so I thought I'd go and investigate. When I got to the man's room I realised he wasn't saying "bear" it was more "bleeurrghh" and he was being sick into a cardboard box just as I got into his room! Daddy shouted at me from across the garden and gave one of his stares—it's very funny when he does that. I don't think he understood what I was doing.

Mummy is very lovely because she knew that me and Millie would really miss her very much so before she went into hospital she bought the three of us some identical little dogs. Mine is called Daisy, Millie's is Maisie and Mummy's is Crazee. The idea is that whenever we miss Mummy too much we can cuddle our little dog and know that Mummy has the same dog she is cuddling at the hospital too. It is a great idea and I've taken Daisy with me everywhere. Every morning Mummy also organises for there to be an envelope on our place mats when we sit down to breakfast. I have no idea how she gets it there when she is in hospital but I expect Daddy is involved somehow. We get a card and a little present. Daddy reads the cards and it must be very difficult for him to read as it always seems to make his eyes water a bit when he reads them to us.

Yesterday we both got water pistols for the bath which were brilliant. Mummy put in the card that it was my job to squirt Daddy lots. They are so powerful I could get him even when he was on the other side of the bathroom. His T shirt was wetter than us by the time we had finished. Daddy thought these were great presents too—he said something like "oh—excellent—water pistols" when we opened them up so I knew straight away what a good present it was.

Everyone at school is being really nice to me and I got upset Tuesday at the start as Daddy didn't put my lunchbox in the right place. Mrs Overbury and Mrs Burgess both gave me a cuddle and it was OK. Later in the day Mrs Pinn told me we should do a painting of Daisy to take to Mummy. Mrs Pinn did the outline and I did the painting.

Mummy has put it on her door and says she thinks it is really good. The school were very good Mrs Burgess even made sure I had blu-tack with me so we could put it up straight away.

We can't wait for Mummy to come home and I think she will be happy to be home too. Daddy, Millie and I watered all her plants and vegetables so she will be pleased. Mind you the naughty rabbits could be in trouble as they have eaten all her cabbages—it will end up being because Daddy didn't do something he should have I expect.

Me and Millie want you to know that we are missing Mummy though. I cry at the times when I'm used to her being there the most—like at the start and end of school and when I go to bed. Daddy says it's a good thing to cry and he just hugs me. Last night I wanted him to pray that Mummy would be well enough to come home on Friday without her bottle and tube. And so we did and then I cried for quite a long time and I think Daddy probably did too. He said he didn't but he had to blow his nose and I felt a tear drop onto my pyjama top so I know he did really—he was just too embarrassed to admit it. Like I've said—he is silly sometimes.

Anyway that's all our news. Me and Millie have to go now because I've got to get to school and Millie wants to play a Mr Tumble game. She can get very stroppy if she doesn't get her own way. You know what these toddlers are like don't you.

Lots of love

Rose x

PS Daddy always tells me how many people have read his blog so please forward this on to lots of your friends so they read it. It would be soooo funny if I got more people reading my blog than he gets for his. Thanks!!

41

Legacy of a Dad

Well goodness me this has been quite a week!

Miranda is now home and looking amazing as ever (and it's not just me who has said that by the way!). She arrived home from hospital on Friday morning as planned. Of course, understandably, she still is in a little discomfort but her only pain relief is paracetamol and her body reminds her if she overdoes things (this is inevitable with Miranda). Yesterday morning she made it to ballet but then had a two hour sleep whilst the girls and I did the usual Saturday morning shop in Fram. Today she has been to Church, cooked Sunday lunch, having harvested her broad beans and peas from the garden, entertained the girls and helped put them to bed. She is incredibly strong.

Once more I need to use this blog to record my thanks to all of you who have read the posts over the past week. Your support and messages via the comments section as well as through cards, texts, emails, phone calls, Facebook messages, Twitter feeds has been overwhelming and has paid a large part in keeping us going. Aside from the messages we have continued to receive food parcels, flowers and visits. To say thank you doesn't seem adequate to express how we both appreciate all that has been done for us. I shan't pretend this has been a fantastic week but it is behind us and we so value all of you who have, in some way, "walked" with us. I'm sorry that I haven't been able to respond to every message individually but I hope you realise that they meant a lot.

So next week starts with a familiar theme to it. Tomorrow I have to take Miranda to the hospital for her regular Herceptin treatment which was delayed from last Wednesday but once that is done then it is back to work for me and we can establish more of a familiar routine. Miranda's sister Lou is arriving which will be perfect. There is no one better than an older sister, who happens to also be a nurse, to ensure that Miranda takes it easy and doesn't overdo things. I'm happy to pass that baton of responsibility over for a few days!

Of course it's been Fathers Day today so this morning I was able to enjoy opening my cards from Rose and Millie. Rose had made me a tile at Rainbows (pre-Brownies group) and Millie settled for jumping on me in the bed landing with both heels straight on my most sensitive area. So painful and I'm still walking rather gingerly this evening. Happy Fathers Day! The tile from Rose was great—they were apparently told to paint pictures on the tiles of things their Daddy liked best. Rose decided for me that meant football, cricket, coffee and rainbows—with some flowers and hearts thrown in to show she loves me. Very sweet and, of course, I'm so proud of it.

Rose even told me that the coffee she has drawn is my favourite Paddy & Scotts "Great with Friends" variety which, whilst difficult to discern from the drawing, is still spot on for accuracy!

Now the fun of choosing, writing and giving a card for Father's Day has been denied me for the last four years. I lost my Dad thanks to a stroke in 2007, a year before our youngest daughter was born. I think, strangely, Fathers Day somehow takes on more meaning when you don't have a Dad as well as the more obvious poignancy that is added to the day. Rose's gift to me this morning made me think about what I would have drawn on a tile for my Dad—plenty of sporting themes for him too. Football, cricket and latterly, bowls to be precise. I would probably have drawn some laughter as my Dad was always quick with the one-liners, loved to tease and would love nothing more than watching a bit of comedy on the TV. Problem is—he'd never have worked it out as my artistic skills are already way behind what Rose can do.

Until you lose someone you are really close to I don't think you appreciate how hard it is to deal with that loss. Or the fact that whilst the initial hurt does subside there is a soreness and pain that never goes away. Well at least I never appreciated that. For Mothers Day I posted up a letter I sent to my Mum trying to help her understand the situation with Miranda's illness a little better as she has struggled to come to terms with it. Today I've been pre-occupied with thoughts of what I want my Dad to know. And, courtesy of this virtual world within which this blog lives, as I clearly can't tell him I thought I'd share them with you. I hope you don't mind.

Dear Dad

Well four years on and I still hate the fact I can't send you a Father's Day card. I want you to know that I still miss you as much as ever. It's funny because certain things happen or news breaks, like the fixture lists for the new football season come out, and I find myself thinking "ooh must remember to tell Dad that Ipswich are away on Boxing Day" and then I realise I can't do that anymore. And that still really hurts.

I got my Father's Day cards today from Rose and Millie. You would love both your Grandchildren so deeply. Rose, of course, has changed so much since you knew her. She is such a caring and compassionate little girl. I've worked really hard to keep the memory of you alive for her and I'm so chuffed that she still talks about you a lot, she always wants to go and visit your stone at the cemetery and knows that her Grandpa was very funny and made people smile. She remembers events and things we did with you but I suspect that is more down to us telling her rather than a real recollection but still that's good enough for me.

Of course you never knew Millie, but you need to know that she shares your sense of impish humour and has inherited your sweet tooth. Do you remember how during the last few years you were with us, when your short term memory was fading, you would go to the loo and then get lost trying to find your way back to the sitting room and I'd come and rescue you from the hall somewhere. However all through that time no matter how well Miranda hid away the bars of chocolate in the pantry you would still find them and we would catch you munching on them. We became convinced that you had replaced your memory with a heightened sense of smell! Well Millie has that same ability to seek out chocolate!

When she was born there was more than one person that told us that Millie even looked a lot like you. I almost know what they meant but this is something that we hope for her sake she will grow out of very quickly! In many respects maybe it is good that the two of you never met I think you would have ganged up and got yourselves into so much trouble. She would have loved you so much though and I wish you knew that.

I love being their Dad and as I get more experienced in that role I realise how much I learnt from you. You were simply the best Dad and if my two think half as much of me as I did of you then I'll be pretty proud to be honest. If I was to sum up the stand out memory of how you parented me it would be that you made me feel so special. Your encouragement of all that I did was so crucial in my development and I can honestly say I cannot remember a single time when you got really cross with me. I hope that is because I don't remember much of my first five or so years and not that you didn't get cross with me as a young child otherwise I have already failed to live up to the standards you set!

Dad, I can't pretend that the last six months have been easy and I could have done with you being around more than ever. I so need the encouragement and reassurance that you gave me as I try to find a way through with Miranda and her battle with cancer. If nothing else, you would have helped Mum through this and that would have been one less thing for me to contend with.

But the thing is Dad in the forty two years we shared you were so loving, and most important of all, so consistent in your advice. That consistency means that I can be pretty certain of what you would say now. I know what you would say to Mum and how you would have wanted me to deal with her as well as the life challenges that get thrown at me. I hope you realise that is your greatest legacy. You may not be around to remind me but I can take action with the confidence of your blessing.

I will work hard to create the same legacy for Rose and Millie.

Both of them can throw a strop or two about the most insignificant thing and they both shout "it's not funny" when they are really cross. When they do, I've taught them one of your favourite songs—the one that starts "when you're smiling, when you're smiling, the whole world smiles with you". I remember you singing that to me when I had a tantrum—clearly this became embarrassing by the time I was 27 years old!

Anyway singing that song as I regularly do always reminds me of you so much. There have been quite a few times that the line "but when you're crying, you bring on the rain" could have applied to me over the past few months but, just like you always told me, I make sure the smiling always wins out in the end.

And I really want you to know that. I so hope you do.

Happy Fathers Day!
Dave x

42

Aunty Lou and a Legend

Actually I probably should have called this post—Aunty Lou is a legend—and my two girls certainly wouldn't disagree. Miranda's sister Lou has been with us this week and it has been great for all of us. She went home Friday and regularly throughout the weekend Millie has been asking

"Where's Aunty Lou?"

A sure sign of how much she is being missed already.

Aside from it being great for the girls it has been good for Miranda and I too. Being medically trained Lou has been able to ensure that Miranda has not been overdoing it and the great news is that Miranda continues to recover so well from the operation. Was it really just under two weeks ago? It seems so much longer since she was in hospital. Aside from a swelling under her arm, which will be looked at tomorrow when we go back to see the consultant and get the post-op results, Miranda is doing amazingly well, both physically and emotionally, and that is such a relief.

Lou has done lots of housework and been a great help driving Miranda and the girls around. I think it was probably a good week for Lou too. I know only too well how tough it is to stand on the sidelines and watch someone you are really close to battle with this disease, and for Lou it has been even tougher to do that remotely, living over 150 miles away in Oxford. It must have been so difficult to only be able to know what is going on through phone calls and texts.

So I'm sure Lou enjoyed being able to show her support in a practical, close at hand way—and she did that really well and we all loved having her around—I even got to have at least one glass of wine poured out ready for me every night!

So apart from the legendary Lou, on Friday night I got to meet and spend some time with Sir Garfield Sobers—probably one of the finest cricketers the game has ever known. Indeed such is his prominence that a panel of 100 cricketing experts were asked to vote for the five greatest cricketers of the 20th century and all but 10 picked Sobers. I got to meet him because he came to open my cricket club, Worlingworth's new pavilion, courtesy of a chance meeting in Barbardos between our Club Captain and Sir Garfield. To describe this as a bit of a coup is a massive understatement! A true cricketing legend coming to a Suffolk village which has less than 1,000 inhabitants. Apparently it appealed to him to come and experience a bit of rural English village cricket. So we turned our opening night into a true Caribbean evening with steel band, hog roast and over 250 people turned up. I got to be the master of ceremonies and that afforded me the chance to spend a bit of time with the legend that is Sir Garfield Sobers.

What struck me most about the man was his humility. He was as interested in the people he spoke to as they were in him. He spent time with the youth team players in the nets and, having arrived for the evening purely for the cost of his petrol from London, he then stayed over an hour longer then he originally promised. Moreover his "few words" to mark the opening turned into a full "after dinner" style speech lasting 25 minutes before he opened the floor to take questions. He then spent over an hour signing autographs, patiently having his photograph taken with every autograph hunter. When he left I still got the impression he had enjoyed the evening as much as we had!

Given the behaviour of some of the modern day sporting greats, and their ability to dominate the front as well as the back pages of the newspaper, and the obvious arrogance and disregard they display for others, Sir Garfield left a lasting impression on me. It made me consider what defines true greatness. His sporting record can only leave you in awe—his name litters the record books, he could bat and bowl and who else has a stand named after them while they are still alive? But the thing is, what I will now remember most about him was the way that, despite all his achievements, he was more interested in finding out about others that night than he was in talking about himself. And all this despite the fact that he had some story to tell!

Very few of us, and least of all me, will ever reach the heights of excellence in our chosen field of endeavour that Gary Sobers achieved in his. But how many of us, when given the opportunity to talk about what we do to an eager audience, would demonstrate the sense of humility and interest in others? He was a hugely impressive character and meeting him left me with plenty of food for thought.

It was just the best way to open our new pavilion and ground and the whole evening will live long in the memory. It was great as Miranda was able to come along too, with the girls, which made it into a family night out and we haven't had many of those lately.

So all told you would think we have had a great week, and as I sit out on our patio writing this, listening to John Legend on the CD and drinking Pimms in the late evening Suffolk sunshine, there is so much that has been positive for me to reflect upon. Actually let's be clear, whilst I'm listening to John Legend, Miranda is soaking in the evening bird song which I must confess is an incredible garden soundtrack that we are lucky enough to enjoy.

But I can't close the story of our week without recording that it has also been a really sad week too. One of our friends at the Forge passed away on Wednesday in just the most tragic of circumstances. It is one of those events that when you first hear about, you actually find yourself catching your breath as it seems too much to take in.

Miranda and I didn't know Paul that well, but I had often chatted with him about Compassion, a charity that he was a staunch and active supporter of and which my business is also involved with. He was someone that I was so used to seeing on a Sunday morning and passing the time of day with. And now he has gone. And for his family that must be so incredibly tough to deal with. It is yet one more reminder that no matter how hard life seems to us at the moment there are always others who are going through far worse. So right now my thoughts are occupied by Paul and the wonderful family he has left behind.

The events of this week and my meeting with Sir Garfield have reminded me once more that as we travel through life there are so many everyday experiences which teach us lessons about what is important and what is not.

I just hope I remember to learn from those lessons.

43

Take That and Party!

Never did I think that two little words "complete response" would set my heart racing with excitement. Or that they would metaphorically and physically put a smile on my face, a skip in my step and set my hat at a jaunty angle. But that's exactly what they did today when we went to meet with the consultant to get the results of Miranda's mastectomy.

You see a "complete response" means that the chemotherapy has done its job. When the experts analysed under microscope the tissue and lymph nodes that had been removed from Miranda they found absolutely no trace of any cancer cells. Amazing . . . . they'd gone . . . . disappeared . . . . finished . . . . nuked . . . . killed . . . . take that cancer!

Brilliant!

The consultant explained that when people have chemo before surgery there are three possible responses that can happen when the tissue is analysed. No response means that the chemo hasn't really worked and the cancer has continued to grow throughout the treatment. This is obviously bad news and fortunately a rare occurrence. We already knew that Miranda's tumours had reduced in size so this wouldn't be the result in her case. A partial response is the most common outcome and it means that the chemo has worked but there are a few traces of cancer left in the tissue removed. This is fairly normal and why surgery is carried out to ensure all the cancer is removed. A complete response however means that the chemo was so effective it has removed the cancer entirely. It is the best possible result anyone could hope for. A moment to literally stop and thank God.

Clever old oncologist! Well done chemo! The impact it had on Miranda was pretty grim but it was all worthwhile. Miranda survived. The cancer didn't.

The power of prayer and medicine combined is clearly a potent force and how we have valued both.

When we were told today Miranda just looked at the consultant and said

"I've got goosebumps!"

And I discovered I'd magically swallowed a golf ball and it had got stuck in my throat! I never realised that the chemo could be so completely effective and, of course, I now think the medical researchers need to find a way of removing tissue, analysing it and then, if it gets the all clear, put it back again! I mean, why not?! They can do pretty amazing stuff already can't they?

So what now? Well we drove from the hospital to Fram and called into the Castle pub and Miranda had a Pimms in the sunshine and I had a Shandy!

Of course there is still the small issue of radiotherapy to be undertaken. Five weeks of it, everyday to be precise. The Herceptin treatment will continue every three weeks until Christmas. But then Miranda is on to six month checkups, with mammograms and CT scans, for the next five years. But that's it. She is officially clear of cancer! Woo-hoo!

To complete the good news the swelling on Miranda's arm which had been worrying her turned out to be post-op fluid which the consultant drained off today. She also removed the surgical dressing, thought the wound had healed really well and was impressed at the range of movement that Miranda had in her arm and shoulder joint already. It could not have been better if we had been allowed to write the script!

I've often talked about this being like a mountain climb of a journey that we are on. Well I just think the summit has loomed into view—and it is a very beautiful site.

Now before we get too carried away there remains the same chance of the cancer returning as there has always been but as Miranda said earlier today bring on December 2015! The five year anniversary is quite a target in the survival stakes but today it feels like it all got a bit closer. We've not forgotten our mantra of "expect the unexpected" and there are still the opportunities for so many things to trip us up between now and then, but forgive us a little celebration at what we've learnt today. Take that cancer!

After the meeting with the consultant this afternoon we sat and talked and planned for the months ahead for the first time with a real sense of certainty and conviction about those plans. That felt good. Miranda building her pizza oven in the garden, a family holiday (boy do we feel like we need one of those!) were high on the list. For the immediate term I need to get my lines learnt for a play I'm in on Sunday week (goodness that has crept up on me!) and for Miranda she has a certain concert at Wembley Stadium a week today to look forward to . . . .

Take That and party indeed!

PHASE THREE

THE RADIOTHERAPY

44

The Elephant in the Room

Yesterday was the village Rounders tournament! It was a lovely day and we are so lucky to have people living in our tiny village who are so good at organising such things. So over 80 people attended (this is almost a third of the village population) and over 50 took part in the Rounders. Needless to say, nothing was going to stop Miranda from taking part and it was the type of tournament where it was OK for Millie, our two year old, to make her debut.

Millie is of the age, and I think probably personality, where she is determined to do everything herself. So, whereas Rose wanted any assistance she could get with hitting the ball and even fielding, Millie, after two goes with me helping her to hit the ball, announced "I can do it myself." She stood, bat at shoulder height and ready to hit anything that came in her direction. Each innings was on a timed basis and it just so happened that our innings ended with Millie next to go. The teams swapped over and our players all went out to field except for Millie. The nuances of timing and end of innings were lost on her, she loved to bat and it was her go. A gentle explanation resulted in an emotional breakdown that all 2 year olds specialise in and so the referee wisely announced that we would just let Millie have her bat before starting the next innings.

So the game stopped and everyone watched. The bowler pitched the ball, Millie hardly moved her bat and the ball sailed past her to back stop. Millie set off to first base and then, because this is what she likes to do, just kept running. Spontaneously everyone watching broke out into cheers for Millie and a chant of "rounder . . . . rounder . . . . rounder" went up. And with the biggest grin you can imagine she completed her run around all four bases and got a huge cheer as she finished! It was a kind of "Field of Dreams" moment!

It was very sweet anyway, for me and Miranda, as much as it was for Millie. But I couldn't help thinking isn't it a shame that life is not like that. Wouldn't it be so cool that if things didn't quite go your way, you could just stop the world, push pause, and then recreate an outcome that was much more in line with what we wanted. Imagine if you could live a life where you got a second shot at something if you messed up, rather than the one chance that we actually get. At some point Millie will have to learn that lesson.

The Rounders was a good way to end what has been a good week. After Monday's encouraging news we've enjoyed some champagne and the mood has been pretty upbeat to be honest. Miranda had her regular MUGA heart scan to make sure that the Herceptin treatment is not causing any damage and, whilst at the hospital, had some more fluid drained off from under her arm and met with her oncologist. The expectation is that her radiotherapy will start in the last week of July at the latest.

The radiotherapy feels like the final stage in this journey and once it is concluded then Miranda only has the three weekly Herceptin to contend with. Inevitably I've found myself looking back and questioning how well we have coped so far living with Miranda's cancer. My biggest fear, well one of them anyway, was how the children would deal with it.

Whilst realising that it is far too early to tell the true impact that this episode will have on them I am reasonably pleased at how they seem to be coping to date. I'm not sure there is a right and a wrong way to handle this—it's much more that there is the way that feels most comfortable and that's probably the best way. We have wanted to be really honest with our children and to answer any and every question they have. Fortunately neither of them has ever asked the awkward "will Mummy die?" question. If they do, we have already agreed that we would explain along the lines of, some people who have the illness that Mummy has don't recover but that what we all need to do is keep praying that Mummy will be fine; help Mummy as much as we can; and remember that Mummy is very determined to get better as soon as possible.

Of course this honesty has led to some entertaining moments like the time when Rose, Millie and I were in a coffee shop and Rose got the friendly waitress into conversation which led to her suddenly explaining that "her Mummy was in hospital having one of her boobies taken away". The expression on the waitress's face was priceless—I stepped in to save her having to respond!

I realise it is partly a generational thing but my Mum's view is very much that we tell the girls too much. I remember her being perturbed that we were going to break the news to the girls of Miranda's diagnosis before the Christmas holiday. "Oh at least let them enjoy Christmas first" was her response. We had no idea how we would all cope with Christmas, coming so soon after diagnosis and the first chemo session on Christmas Eve, so it was our view that it was better they knew, than picked up on some unspoken upset or worry.

I still remember when Miranda was first told that there was a moment, when she went through to the waiting room to see the oncologist, where she was so tempted to just run away. It was an understandable emotion and there have been moments too when I've felt the need to escape.

In fact we both would have liked the world to have stopped and people to have allowed us to replay the situation with a much better outcome—something like—"oh actually it's not cancer after all—just a bit of a blocked milk duct in your breast that's all".

Anyway I think what I've come to learn is that all of us, at different times, are likely to face difficult situations or life challenges. And sometimes those situations can become the "elephant in the room". It's big and obvious but we choose not to talk about it because it's difficult or we are not sure what to say—so we ignore it. We carry on with life pretending not to notice this large "elephant" that's moved in with us.

And what I've also realised is that very often the thought of dealing with the situation is so much worse than the reality of actually dealing with it. I remember years ago, way before I met Miranda, that I allowed a situation to develop. I shied away from dealing with it. I ignored the elephant in the room. No matter how much worse things got, and believe me they did, I still kept ignoring it. The outcome was that a few people got very hurt. It cost me a marriage. I messed up big time. If I could have stopped the game I would have replayed it so differently. But of course I couldn't and I have to live with the damage I caused.

It's why this time around I am so determined to face up to this challenge and to deal with whatever is thrown at us. It's why I am so amazed, inspired and even more in love with my wife for the way she has battled this disease. The way she has tackled all that has been thrown at her over the last six months.

And it's partly why I've been writing this blog and will continue to do so over the next few months of treatment. I need you to hold me to account for how I'm supporting my family, how I'm facing up to the elephant in the room. It reminds me of a cliché I learned through business that you tackle huge tasks in the same way that you would eat an elephant—one bite at a time.

And there is a small part of me that hopes, that if there is an elephant in your room right now that our story might offer just a tiny bit of encouragement and hope.

We can fight this you know—just take one bite at a time.

45

Out of Africa

It's been a bit of a strange old week.

For Miranda the highlight has been the visit to Wembley Stadium to see "Take That" or perhaps "That's That" as my Mother innocently refers to them much to my amusement! Miranda had just the best time and the dulcit tones of Gary, Howard, Jason, and Mark have been regularly wafting across our kitchen pretty incessantly over the last few days. Try as I might I just don't share the love for this particular music genre!

On the health front, there continues to be good news. A trip to the consultant to drain off more fluid from her wound was successful and, more importantly, there was much less fluid to drain off which is really encouraging. Her wound is healing remarkably well and, as ever, Miranda is dealing with the whole situation with incredible bravery and humour. She has been sorting out swimming costumes so that she can get back in the pool when her hair has got a bit longer and was quick to point out to me that it is more expensive having one boob rather than two! I was able to enjoy a quick fashion parade of the various costume options and had to confirm that the prosthetic implant was of a suitably matching size. It was something that we were able to have a laugh about and I do think that is the best way to deal with it.

Aside from alternative fashion parades the Courteen household has been busy with preparations for the birthday of the youngest member who turns three tomorrow. Presents have been wrapped, cards written and a chocolate cake has been made with a "Peppa Pig jumping up and down in muddy puddles" icing top that has been painstakingly created by my very clever wife.

Today has been the village fete and we've all had a fun afternoon enjoying the various games and stalls that do typify a traditional English village fete. I met up with a few of my cricket mates and was reminded once more that this journey Miranda and I are on is not one we walk alone. The wife of one of my cricketing friends had breast cancer two years ago and it has now returned . . . . I can only imagine.

This week would also have been the week when Miranda would have travelled to Zambia with a team from our Church—The Forge. She was all booked and planning to go before her diagnosis came through and were it not for her cancer, would have flown out on Tuesday. The Zambia project is one our Church has been involved with for a few years and we partner with Hands at Work who are based over in Africa. The team spend time visiting the poorest of communities and provide basic health care training whilst they are there. Miranda intends to be part of the team next year. So the team flying out this week was a little reminder of how our plans have been changed by cancer.

I can only imagine the profound effect experiencing such poverty close up must have. And I've seen the impact it has had on numerous friends who have already been to Zambia through this project. Oliver is a good friend of mine and he is on the team out there right now that Miranda should have been part of. He is writing a blog about his trip but this morning's post was so amazing—the story it tells so incredible—that I felt compelled to share it with you here.

He called his post "It's Not Alright Said Fred" and here is what Oliver wrote:

> *Fred is a man of peace. He's special. I've had the privilege of walking and talking with Fred today and I'll never forget it.*
>
> *Fred was the headmaster of the village school we visited he's not been paid, but cares for the people in his community in a way that I've not experienced before.*
>
> *Fred's community is poor, the people originally moved to the area to work in the nearby copper mine, but when that closed they were left to survive, literally. There is no clean water. There's not enough food, there is no money. I'd describe it as desperate. Fred wouldn't.*
>
> *Fred paints a picture of a better future, he thanks God for the support he has had to help him support his community members better. He knows that the future will be better than the past. And his life is a testament to it.*
>
> *Just a couple of years ago Fred would have died if it were not for the changes in international policy that now provides HIV medication for free. He's recovered and because of that his whole community is benefiting from the hope that he brings them. He's been in it and remains in it for the long haul.*
>
> *Romans 5:3 could have been written for (or even by) Fred.*
>
> *"We can rejoice when we run into trials because we know that they bring endurance. Endurance develops strength of character, and*

character develops our confident hope in salvation. This hope won't lead to disappointment, because we know that God loves us dearly"

So "it's not alright" said Fred. He's not happy with the way things are, but you won't hear him grumble because he's too busy doing something about it.

So powerful. Puts into context what we have experienced over the past six months. I'm amazed at Fred's story. And I hope my amazing wife, Miranda, gets to meet him one day too.

46

Winners and Losers

Goodness me I can't believe it has been two weeks since I last posted. Clearly last weekend flew by as I was having a go at parenting solo whilst Miranda went back to her parents for her orchestra weekend. A full two days of cello playing culminating in a two hour concert in the Stratford Civic Hall on the Sunday night. She had a great time and her arm and fingers survived the onslaught. Amazing, given that it is only just over a month since her operation.

The girls and I had fun too but the weekend reminded me that I do not understand how single parents cope and, once more, they have my utmost respect. I headed into work on Monday, after the school and nursery drop, absolutely shattered!

The last fortnight has included the usual hospital trips for Miranda as they prepare her for the radiotherapy, which starts this coming Wednesday, and her regular dose of Herceptin.

It has been a bit of a sporting week too what with the Open Golf Championship last weekend and . . . . errrmmm . . . . well Rose's sports day too! I was able to sneak away from work to attend her first ever sports day. I'm so very grateful that Rose's school adhere to the traditional form of sports day with running races, egg and spoon races and the like with stickers and certificates for the winners. I think that is so, so important.

There are many schools these days that have ditched this in favour of some new fangled games which are creative but don't have winners and losers. The theory being that it is unfair to allow children to be losers! I think that is really misguided. Life is full of winners and losers and we are all likely to experience both at different times. School is about preparing us for life and sports day is the first opportunity some children have to experience these emotions. A great chance for them to learn how to win with humility and lose with dignity. I'd briefed Rose beforehand that if she lost she had to go up to the winner and say "well done". She remembered, bless her, but only had to do this once in the four races she was in, as in the other three she was the winner! That's my girl!

Of course there was a race for parents too. I was a little disappointed that the Dads only had a sack race—this is not my speciality. It at least gave me the opportunity to experience losing with dignity! Although the way I lurched over the line at the end to claim 4th place didn't actually demonstrate much dignity to be fair. I was so determined to beat one of Rose's best friend's . . . . Granddad! Phew—close call that one!

Miranda, of course, did the Mum's sack race too. And, of course, she won it—inevitable really. She didn't tease me about this very much at all?!

Back to the Open Golf and I managed to persuade Millie and Rose to allow me to watch the last few holes on the Sunday as the tournament reached its conclusion. Millie wasn't really interested but Rose tried to understand what was going on and amused me greatly when she announced that her teacher at school was very good at golf.

"Let's look closely Daddy, Mrs Burgess is probably playing in this"!

Probably not actually Rose.

Like many people I was pleased that Darren Clarke won. I mean in how many other sports can a "40 something" win one of the biggest tournaments? Even snooker and darts seem to be won by younger competitors these days. After the disappointment of the sack race here was some hope for me.

But it not just the fact that we are in the "forty somethings" bracket that links me with Darren Clarke. We also share the fact that we have experienced our wives suffering from breast cancer. This was alluded to regularly over the last few holes as Clarke closed in on victory with the commentators making reference to the fact that "he's been through such tough times—he deserves this" and comments such as "this will be such a popular victory after all he's been through." And they were very true of course.

As I watched I couldn't help reflecting the long term impact cancer has on your life. It does seem to mean that whatever happens subsequently, cancer becomes a reference point. I was so impressed at the way that Darren Clarke humbly accepted his trophy and at the way he talked about his wife in his acceptance speech. And I was equally impressed that he partied all night to celebrate too! But I couldn't help wonder if he wouldn't prefer his victory to have been referenced by something other than the loss of his wife to breast cancer? Wouldn't he prefer that the amazing consistency he showed over the 4 rounds of the championship was the talking point? Or by the fact that having been ranked in the top 4 golfers in the world his game slipped away completely but he went away, reinvented his game and, at 42, came back to win his first major?

I think the point I'm trying to make here is this. Before Miranda had cancer I would have been just like the commentators. I'd have gone into work on Monday morning and would have talked about how great it was Darren Clarke won the Open after losing his wife to cancer. And I think that's because we all have this natural fear of the disease and how we would deal with it. When that fear becomes reality it somehow shrinks in size. It just becomes part of everyday life. It's really rubbish but you just deal with it, you have no other choice of course. Cancer is no longer the same big deal and the fact that people referred to it in the context of Darren Clarke's win brought home to me, for the first time probably, the change in mindset I've gone through.

Those of you who watched the last round of the golf will know that the only time that Clarke's victory was in doubt was when Phil Mickelson mounted a surge in the middle of his round. The poignancy here is that Darren Clarke's wife had breast cancer, recovered and spent two years in remission before it returned and claimed her life in 2006. Phil Mickelson's wife was diagnosed with the same disease in 2009 and Clarke has been actively supporting the couple through it. Mickelson's wife is currently in remission. Clarke held on to win the Open this time.

Made me think—just as I'd explained to Rose—in life we all get to experience winning and losing.

47

Tattoos

My wife came home last week and announced that she had got three tattoos done. Permanent ones. Ones that will be with her for the rest of her life. I was shocked to be honest. I mean whilst I realise that tattoos are far more commonplace these days, and indeed some of my best friends and closest family members have them, I just don't get them. I can't see the point. So I was slightly unnerved that my wife should go and get three without even consulting me!

My mind raced to all sorts of images of butterflies, hearts or our children's names in Hebrew or something. And where might these tattoos be I pondered!

Anyway I needn't have worried the tattoos are just dots—three of them strategically placed on her upper body to help with the radiotherapy—to make sure that they zap her in exactly the right place. And today she gets "zapped" for the first time! A daily occurrence for the next five weeks. She had some large crosses on her upper body too but these will eventually wear off—the dots are proper tattoos and they are here to stay. One more forever reminder of this disease as if we needed it.

It got me thinking about how I would react if my children grew up and decided to get a tattoo. I had a friend with a teenage daughter who had a rather large number of piercings and studs in places that were very visible and not so visible—apparently! I loved his attitude which was along the lines of

"I'd much prefer it if she didn't have all the studs but I'm not going to let a little bit of ironmongery get in the way of our relationship!"

I hope I develop the same level of empathy if necessary with my daughters but who knows? It is quite a few years away yet—thankfully!

Now of course the last couple of days the newspapers have been full of someone who famously was covered in numerous tattoos. The death of Amy Winehouse has provoked a huge amount of coverage in the national press and through social media sites such as Twitter and Facebook. It has been a pretty diverse reaction. There have been many tributes to someone who possessed such an amazing talent. In contrast, there have also been a number of comments critical of her and the amount of attention given to her death in comparison with the coverage over the loss of a British soldier fighting in Afghanistan.

Now let me be clear; I am horrified at the scale of the losses our armed forces are experiencing in a war that I don't really understand the purpose of, and to which there appears to be no imminent end. But I think it is impossible to compare the value of the loss of one life over another, irrespective of how that life was lived or lost. And as for the media coverage—well that will always be determined by what sells the newspapers.

For me, the death of Amy Winehouse was a real tragedy. It was such a waste of a talented individual. I enjoyed her music. She had an incredible voice, wrote great songs and her lyrics gave us, at times, a piercing insight into the struggles she faced. I am so sad that she never lived to fulfil her potential and I am sad for all the great songs that will now never get written. I guess the degree to which you feel empathy towards her will be dependent upon whether you liked her music and whether you believe addiction is a behaviour we choose or an illness. For me it is most definitely the latter.

I've only ever experienced addiction at close hand on two occasions. Both were in individuals who were members of gyms I worked in. And both became addicted to exercise—it happened right before my eyes. A healthy habit became an unhealthy behaviour pattern. Their lives suddenly revolved around getting their next exercise fix to the complete detriment of family, work and social life. They were perfectly normal, sensible people who just got addicted to the endorphins that are released into our brains when we exercise. And nothing any of us did could get them to stop. We had to wait until the individuals concerned recognised and accepted they had a problem.

That's why addiction is so horrible. It reminds me a little of cancer. Cancer lives inside us, attacking our body until our body can cope no more or until the chemo gets to it. Addiction lives in our mind and causes behaviour that is irrational and damaging until our body can cope no more or until our mind "gets" what is happening.

I'm genuinely not sure there was much Amy Winehouse alone could have done about her addiction and that is what makes her loss so tragic. Now I know nothing really about the person that Amy was beyond what we saw in the media. She certainly seemed from the moment she entered the public eye to have a certain vulnerability about her personality. Her life seemed to spiral out of control when she became involved with the guy who ultimately became her husband for a while. She could perhaps have chosen her friends more carefully.

But the person who has been in my thoughts so much over the last few days has been her Dad, Mitch Winehouse. Being a Dad of girls myself I'm bound to have a natural empathy with him. How tough must his life be right now? Over the past few years I have admired the way he has tried to intervene and help his daughter. A few years ago he faced a certain degree of ridicule by the popular press as the reactionary, controlling father when he publicly expressed his concern over her relationship with Blake Fielder-Civil. I hope I'd be strong enough to do the same if I was ever in that position. According to all reports, he never gave up trying to get Amy to face up to her addiction. And I'm haunted by that interview he gave a few years ago admitting his greatest fear is that her addiction would kill her.

Faced with a helpless situation he never gave up and now that his greatest fear has come true he was among the first to pay glowing tribute to all that was good about his daughter. Just as a great Dad should do.

So last Saturday, the day of Amy Winehouse's death, I did what I do every night before I go to bed, I went to check on my girls. Millie's a light sleeper so I only ever dare spend a moment or two to check she's under the duvet but Rose sleeps more deeply so I allowed myself time just watching her sleep. I wondered about what challenges and awkward situations or friendships would befall her when she became older and how it seemed incredulous that she could ever contemplate damaging herself through drink or drugs. And I wondered if 21 years ago Mitch Winehouse looked at 6 year old Amy and thought the same thing. I guess he probably did. So I found myself praying. I prayed that both my girls would find friends that supported and uplifted them, helped them achieve all they are capable of achieving. I prayed that God would give them discernment over the people they came to trust and spend time with. I've prayed that prayer before but it suddenly had so much more meaning that night because, beyond praying for them, I'm not sure there is much more I can do about their choice of friends.

As I came back downstairs I realised that I'm actually not that bothered about whether my girls get tattoos. There are a number of far more important things to get worked up about. I mean, when you analyse it, the friends we choose can leave far more indelible marks on us than a bit of colourful paint injected into our skin ever can.

Just ask Mitch Winehouse.

48

Hopes and Dreams

So we are in August already. How did that happen? I just seemed to blink and we are suddenly in the eighth month of the year. August is renowned for two things—it's the start of the football season and it's the time of the year when the media are struggling for stories so we can expect bizarre and weird stories to make it into the headlines.

Today is actually the first day of the new football season—well it is if your team is in the Football League. I realise that statement invites goading and banter from any budgie (Norwich) fans who have gloriously returned to the Premiership this year which starts a week later. My team, Ipswich, are in the Championship and so today marks the day when every team in the league set out with hopes and dreams of a successful season. For every fan there is the hope of play-offs or promotion tinged with the realism of knowing that for a few teams this will be the first day of a relegation campaign. At least Ipswich got off to a good start with a 3—0 away win at Bristol City. I've been a fan too long though to get carried away by one result—let's see where we are by the year end!

We can have our hopes and dreams though can't we?

I've also been reading about another game of football that took place a long way from Ashton Gate in Bristol. It was in Uganda in fact. One of our friends, Helen, has been over there for a week with her teenage son and daughter, and a bunch of people from the Possibilities charity, helping to build an extension to a school. As part of the last day some of the team from England got involved with playing a game of football with the local team. Helen's blog has been a fantastic read and gave me the title for this post.

It is a powerful story of hopes and dreams.

I've had a particularly busy week with work. We have three new spas all opening within two weeks of each other at the beginning of September. So there is lots to be done and therefore early starts, much driving and a scary feeling that I'm not quite up to the pace right now. On one of my early morning drives down the M11, I was listening to 5 Live on the radio and they were reporting as headline news a sports reporter who had seen a disc like UFO flying near Stansted Airport that morning. Clearly a slow news day. As part of the story they were interviewing some "UFO expert" who was claiming that he has substantial proof that the British army now has the technology (obtained from a captured alien spacecraft) to fly to the stars and connect with aliens. He was serious and this was August 1st not April 1st. I'm not sure I share his conviction that this is true—I mean, if it was, surely Rupert Murdoch and his dubious reporters would have hacked the odd phone or two and unearthed this major development in technology wouldn't they?

But as I drove past Stansted Airport and saw the huge aircraft taking off and flying above me carrying people to all part of the world I couldn't help thinking about my 5 Live friend, and his amazing technological theories, and comparing that with what Helen, Jack and Zoe were experiencing right now. It struck me that we fly people all around this world, we can send people to the moon and back, but we struggle to feed and provide basic education to millions of people just a continent away. Isn't that just a little bit mad?

Same world—very different hopes and dreams.

Back home, Miranda continues to have her daily dose of radiotherapy. The actual blast of radiotherapy takes less than 5 minutes but the process of getting her prepared and in position means it requires a round trip to the hospital of about 2 hours. It is a big chunk out of the day and the girls are getting used to visiting a different friend every morning whilst this happens. We are so lucky to have so many friends who have willingly volunteered to help out in this way and support us. We hope that this process will ensure that all chance of the cancer returning will be removed. It is designed to remove all traces of any cancer, especially in her neck where the operation was not able to reach. She is a third of the way through now—just the seventeen sessions to go!

And it's made me think about where we were exactly a year ago. Rose was getting ready to start school and now she has a successful first year behind her, I was trying to find new investment for my business which is now in place, and Miranda had just been given the all clear from a mammogram and MRI scan, the threat of breast cancer had been lifted—or so we thought. You never know what's ahead of you do you?

It remains the same world—but we've very different hopes and dreams.

49

Where Have All the Leaders Gone?

This weekend sees another milestone passed for Miranda. She is now halfway through the radiotherapy part of her treatment plan. Thirteen down, twelve to go to be precise. The expected tiredness that this treatment creates is starting to have an effect although Miranda does wonder whether the tiredness is more due to the fact that both children are at home for the school holidays rather than the radiotherapy! I guess we will never know.

The last week has been great as Miranda's sister Lou, her husband Julian and their two gorgeous daughters Chloe and Sophie have been to stay. Our two girls love spending time with their cousins and so everyone has had a great few days and I feel like I've missed out being at work! It's reminded me that we need to ensure Rose and Millie get the chance to grow up with their cousins and, given that they only live just under three hours away, we need to plan in more visits to see them. I'm lucky enough to have a great cousin but Bev and I lived over five hours apart throughout our childhood and therefore only met up at Christmas and once in the summer holiday. We didn't really grow up together and it's only in more recent years that we have had more contact. I don't want it to be the same for Rose and Millie with their cousins.

Anyway the Antonen family left on Wednesday and it's been a bit flat since then to be honest. Miranda has had a small health issue unrelated to her cancer and it is funny how actually she finds these smaller, insignificant issues much harder to deal with in many ways than the cancer itself. It's like every effort has gone into fighting the disease and she has no reserves left.

Now, as you know, this blog sets out to tell the story of our journey through Miranda's battle with breast cancer but the events of the past week have been so significant that I feel compelled to comment on them. The major cities of the UK have seen a level of rioting combined with destruction and looting, unparalleled in my lifetime. I can't claim that we have been directly involved but I did travel through London on Monday evening and watched in amazement as trains were being cancelled due to the violence leaving me very grateful to still be able to escape to Suffolk. I also spent two nights making a few calls to make sure that staff at our health clubs and spas got home safely. None of our businesses were damaged but one of our Manchester spas shut for 48hours as guests didn't fancy taking the risk of entering the city centre.

I think the unnerving factor about these riots has been the fact that they have no real cause or purpose. It's simply wanton violence and a level of personal greed through looting that seems to be at the root of the troubles. The vast number of gangs and the sheer spread of the violence meant the police were outnumbered and unable to respond quickly enough to the many locations where trouble was breaking out. Watching the events unfurl via live news feeds on TV and through social media sites such as Twitter was compelling and disturbing in equal measure.

Over the last few days I've been trying to work out how we have ended up in such a place. A number of commentators have talked about the inequity in society and the fact that these youngsters have nothing and are so disenfranchised with the life they lead. There may be an element of truth in that but the problem is, as the rioters have gradually been appearing in court and sentenced, we've learnt that this wasn't a riot by the unemployed. Teachers, council workers, sales people, insurance agents, fashion models, semi-professional footballers and even soldiers have all been convicted of rioting and looting. Hardly disenfranchised and living in poverty in those professions.

Many Facebook statuses were posted in the immediate aftermath suggesting we send the rioters to Afghanistan "to serve alongside our soldiers to see how brave they really were". As it transpired some of the rioters had actually already done that, they were actually those very same brave soldiers. For me that was a really chilling fact—this really was anarchy in the UK.

We seem to have become a society where we judge success by what we have and not by who we are. We all seem to crave a flat screen TV or the latest trainers or outfit irrespective of how we came about acquiring it. The stories of people at the shop entrances shouting out their orders for goods to the looters inside and of the teenager walking into a trashed jewellers shop and asking the owner who was surveying his devastated business if there was a pair of Raybans left he could have are just beyond belief.

We seem oblivious to the fact that the most important things in life aren't actually "things". What we have experienced this year as a family has been a harsh reminder of the undeniable truth of that cliché.

For me one of the biggest problems we face is a complete lack of good leadership. In a tiny way I've experienced being a leader of our business for over 20 years. I'm still learning and I'm still making mistakes. Leadership is an art not a science. You can't follow a formula but you probably do need to get three things right. You need to provide a vision, you need to demonstrate integrity and you need to be good at communicating the key messages.

So who do people look up to? Who provides our nation with leadership? If you look to the sporting heroes you won't find a great deal of integrity especially in football. Contracts ignored to get the next best deal, the captain of the national team sleeps with his team mates partner. It is all about looking after yourself. I couldn't help smiling at Rio Ferdinand tweeting to the effect that he couldn't understand why people were rioting in their own cities. Of course you can't Rio, when you are on £150,000 a week you buy flat screen TV's out of small change so you don't need to loot shops. People are doing this because they aspire to lifestyle so publicly lived out by Rio and his mates.

In business, the culture of everyone for himself is epitomised by the banking industry which has brought the nation to its knees and the world into recession through chasing the next big deal to earn the individual bonuses. It has all been about the short term and the here and now. Not much vision or integrity to be found here I'm afraid.

With government there has been the expenses scandal. Almost every MP was guilty of fiddling his expenses claim to increase his personal wealth. The PM at the time, Gordon Brown, and the current incumbent, David Cameron, were among those found to have broken the rules.

The media which shapes our thoughts and communicates the main messages of the world in which live has been exposed as using the most unscrupulous of methods to get stories and, when they lack sufficient credible evidence for a story they want to print, they make the rest up anyway. Despite this they wield such power that politicians will still try to woo them and the police will take payments from them to pass on confidential information. The level of corruption has been staggering. The lack of integrity amongst the leaders of these three key institutions could not be more stark.

So given this backdrop perhaps we shouldn't have been so shocked at the riots. In terms of helping yourself when opportunity presents itself the affluent and the powerful amongst us had already got there, way before the looters showed up last week. In the harsh world in which many live in our towns and cities they were just following the example society's leaders have set us.

There is hope in every situation and the response of groups of people turning up with brooms to clear up after the riots, organising collections for those who had lost everything in the fires, all co-ordinated through websites and social media, was so heart warming. Now here was a group of people being mobilised for the common good. Here at local level were a few individuals showing great leadership—there was a clear vision, excellently communicated and delivered with integrity. Let's hope a few people in power learn a lesson or two from this example.

I was beginning to wonder where all the leaders had gone.

50

Fashion Statement

One of the great things over the past few weeks is that Miranda's hair has been growing back to such an extent that she can consider finally going "wigless". As strange as it may seem but I think she has actually got attached to the wig and, as much as she worried about it at first, it has now taken on the role of a kind of adult "security blanket". So to suddenly discard it, is tougher for her than the rest of us might imagine.

I think it is also fair to say the wig has been a good choice—I've lost count of the number of people who have complimented her on her hairstyle whilst clearly oblivious to the fact that she is wearing a wig. The lady in the lingerie shop where Miranda went for her special, post mastectomy fitting was so sure it was real hair she told Miranda she didn't recognise her as her hair had grown! She was partially correct of course but was actually referring to the wig not the real hair underneath that she'd never seen! It's also got to the point where, when I see photos of Miranda with her original, long, pre chemo hair; it looks almost odd. I will admit to finding the wig still a little unnerving although this is mainly due to experiences when Miranda is not actually wearing it. You see just after the wig has been washed Miranda leaves it overnight on its stand on the floor of the shower. My heart still misses a beat every time I enter the bathroom; it's like walking into the scene of a horror movie. I'm convinced she leaves it facing the way it does on purpose. I can't see the stand, just the back of the wig, thus guaranteeing she can enjoy watching me have that split second "stop dead in my tracks moment" every time.

So the big question is when does she go wigless? A hair appointment has been made for mid September and Miranda has decided she needs to have it coloured before it is given a public outing. I think I may have mentioned in earlier blogs that it has, ahem, grown back a little more grey than she would like? Of course the style is important and as well as consulting her hairdresser Miranda has also been taking note of advice from others in a similar position.

A while ago a spa industry friend pointed me in the direction of a blog written by a beauty editor who has also been diagnosed with breast cancer. The blog is called Sophie Feels Better and it has been slightly uncanny to follow Sophie's story as the similarity to Miranda's situation has been amazing. They were diagnosed in the same month, had to have chemo first before a mastectomy and lymph node removal, couldn't have immediate reconstruction and are now on radiotherapy.

I've found it really helpful to follow Sophie's story and Miranda has got into the blog more recently too. It is a brilliant blog and has focussed on how Sophie has tried to look good through the various stages of cancer—it's what you'd expect I suppose from a leading beauty industry journalist—and as she has just ventured out "sans wig" her recent posts have been really relevant. The general message seems to be to focus on the eyes to detract attention from the very short hair. So with Miranda wearing glasses, she has been encouraged by Sophie's blog, and by her friend Bridget (bit of a style guru too!), to think of glasses as a fashion accessory rather than a necessary aid to vision. Make the glasses a fashion statement in fact.

So with Bridget in tow Miranda headed off to the opticians to order a new pair of glasses ready for the new look. She came home and was clearly priming me for a dramatic change to her current pair. By the time she had finished describing how dramatically different these glasses would be all I could think of was Elton John in the early 80⊠s as he went through his Crocodile Rock period. The zanier the better for Elton if you recall!

Anyway yesterday I was whisked into the opticians to give my approval and, whilst I'm sure Elton would have been rather unimpressed, I thought they looked great and am looking forward to the "Miranda Autumn look"!

In fact there is so much to look forward to—Miranda has only 7 more radiotherapy sessions to go, some holidays are just around the corner and this whole cancer journey is feeling more behind us than in front of us. And "I'm still standing" as old Elton might say . . . . wearing a slightly different pair of glasses to those worn by my wife.

Fashion statement indeed!

51

Oxygen Masks

Remember that moment when you're on a plane and the crew go through the safety procedures? There is a bit where they say something like "in the unlikely event that we lose cabin pressure oxygen masks will fall down in front of you. Those of you with children please fit your own mask first".

I haven't taken my girls on a flight yet but every time I hear them go through that part of the message it always makes me think how counter-intuitive that must be. I hope I'm never in that position but I can't imagine I would find it easy putting my mask on first—I'd feel almost compelled to make sure my children were OK before I worried about myself.

But then some things in life are just like that aren't they? We do occasionally need to be counter-intuitive. Of course I understand why they say what they do—by putting your own mask on first you are guaranteed to be in a better position to help your children than if you try to put their masks on first and pass out before you can get your own supply sorted.

I was reminded of the whole oxygen mask briefing this week as I've had the last week off work. I went to amend my auto-response on my work email so that people are aware I'm on holiday and realised that the last time I'd done this was last October! I was amazed—I've gone just eight weeks short of a full calendar year without taking a proper holiday off work. No wonder I've been feeling worn out lately!

Now obviously I have had some days off work but these have been around Miranda's treatment, largely to be with her on her chemo days and also around her mastectomy and other hospital stays. Looking back I can see how it has happened—I've been saving holidays in case Miranda had a prolonged spell in hospital or where she was really ill and I needed to take a chunk of time off but, fortunately, that never really happened and so I've just kept going.

Worse still this wasn't the greatest of weeks to have taken as holiday anyway as we are just about to open 3 spas including one that opens this coming Wednesday and so, understandably, I have had to field the odd enquiry and sort some issues out via phone and email. It has not therefore felt like a "proper holiday" but this week was the most convenient to fit with others who have helped look after the girls whilst Miranda has her radiotherapy. Of course we've not been away because of the daily treatments but I've had some fun taking the girls swimming and we've had the odd afternoon out. This weekend we headed up to the in laws and Miranda and I managed to grab 24 hours on our own at a lovely hotel and spa in Cheltenham. Boy did I need that time out to chill!

The 24 hour spa break also led to the first public "wigless" outing for Miranda. Steam rooms and hydrotherapy pools don't really go with wigs to be honest. I had visions that if she kept her wig on and the hydrotherapy jets came on unexpectedly her wig could be sent across the pool with guests scattering in every direction thinking a small furry animal had escaped and was swimming across the pool! The whole experience went well, Miranda's hair is long enough to not shock anyone or attract any second looks. Indeed most of the odd looks were reserved for me at dinner in the evening when we met the same guests who had been in the spa earlier. I'm sure some of them were convinced I'd spent the afternoon in the spa with one woman and then was taking another to dinner! Amazing how a wig can completely change your appearance!

Incredibly the radiotherapy treatment is nearly complete—just two more sessions to go. As with everything to do with this disease and its treatment programme Miranda has coped amazingly well and better than we hoped. Her skin is now quite pink, a little sore and she is a bit tired but she has been able to carry on with life pretty much as she would have wanted to. She is incredible. Indeed the symptom that bothers her most right now is the regular hot flushes which are a delayed result of the chemotherapy potentially tipping her body into an early menopause. We won't know for certain if this is the case for another eight months or so but we have been told that it is highly unlikely we will be able to have any more children. Good job we planned to quit at two anyway!

So when I look back and review what I've learnt from this journey with cancer I will remember the importance of taking care of myself. In order to best support my wife and children I need to be refreshed and ensuring my batteries are recharged and I've failed to do that so far. I spent so much time worrying about how Miranda and the girls were coping I forgot to ask myself the same question and now I'm running out of energy.

I need to pay more attention to the girl at the front of the plane in the uniform. Please excuse me but I need to go and put this elastic behind my ears, pull the tube towards me and breathe deeply. They are pretty important these oxygen masks aren't they!

Oh yeah—and fit your own first won't you—however counter-intuitive that might feel.

52

Felli Celli Time

Do you ever play that game where you are in a restaurant and try to guess the connection between the groups of people on other tables? No?! Oh—it's just me then. At those Christmas work parties where various businesses take their staff I spend most of the evening working out the profession of the people on the surrounding tables. To be honest I'm not bad at guessing and usually wait until the end of the evening, when most people are drunk, before I go across and ask them what job they do to see if I've guessed correctly. It's true—I don't get out that much . . .

Anyway the preamble is to explain that this weekend we have had an absolute houseful. It has been such a laugh. Eight of Miranda's friends arrived on Friday and have just left—the house suddenly seems almost eerily quiet. The food, including a monster barbecue last night, has been amazing. But if we had not stayed in and gone out to a restaurant instead, I defy anyone to have played my guessing game and got the connection between our group correct. You see there is George, he's a music producer who has worked with the Opera Babes, Blur and Boy George to name but a few; Liz who is retired and has a member of her family who trained as an astronaut; David, who knocks out tunes on his guitar at will and who is so creative he always makes us something beautiful out of wood as a gift—this year was a vase; Judith, retired like Liz, and who like Miranda is fully signed up member of the breast cancer club; John, who works in defence and has an off-the-wall sense of humour; another David, another retiree, whose family own a stunning mill in Worcestershire which is only accessible by boat; Marie-Claire who is a professional gardener and who always provides valuable advice for us as well as being adored by our eldest daughter; and finally "X"—whose job is so top secret that she has to have a pseudonym for a Facebook profile!

And what connects them all with each other and my wife is . . . . the cello! Along with Miranda, and a couple of others, they form the cello section in the Stratford-upon-Avon Symphony Orchestra which Miranda has played in since she was 12. They all meet up to play their cellos and every year have a weekend of playing in our barn. They've named their group the "Felli Celli" and the weekend concludes with a concert at the house of the brother of one of the Davids. The music ranges from the Bond theme, Teddy Bears Picnic and some of their own compositions to more traditional, classical cello pieces. Let me tell you, as a non-musician, there is a beautiful richness to the sound of nine cellos being played that even a tone deaf numpty like me can discern.

Rose, Millie and I become interested spectators to the whole weekend. We do our own thing for some of the time, listen a little and join in with the fun and laughter even though some of the banter and musical discussion goes right over our heads. There was a debate on Friday about the composer Mahler—very difficult cello parts in his orchestral works apparently. And every group of people have another group that is the butt of their jokes don't they. Like Ipswich Town fans might banter about Norwich City fans so cellists banter about the viola players! Who knew?!

We all have that hobby or activity that gets right into the sweet spot of who we are. For Miranda it is playing the cello. She comes alive when she's playing it and I love seeing that. And I enjoy gate crashing the house party of a really wonderful group of people from such varied walks of life who are all linked together by their love of cello playing.

For Miranda this is one of her favourite weekends of the year and it was perfectly timed as she completed her radiotherapy on Wednesday. It was the perfect way for her to celebrate reaching yet another milestone in her recovery. Aside from the Herceptin, and the not insignificant matter of her reconstructive operation in a years time, she is almost at the end of her journey. The radiotherapy has been relatively easy to deal with in comparison to the chemotherapy although it is having a bit of a sting in the tail. Her neck and chest area has gone from a pink to a deep red colour and the skin around her neck is also starting to peel, like a bad case of sunburn. This is a common occurrence in such circumstances, and whilst the treatment may have finished, Miranda has been warned that the effects continue for another two weeks after her final session so her skin may get worse before it gets better.

One of the rather obvious but nonetheless important lessons this cancer experience has taught us is that no matter how urgent "stuff" may be there is nothing more important than making sure you allocate time to do the things you really love to do, and spend time with the people you really love spending time with. This weekend Miranda got to do both which is great, and no more than she deserves after all she has gone through this year.

What the cello is to Miranda so the cricket bat is to me! This weekend has reminded me that although this season, for obvious reasons, has passed by without me donning the whites, next year I am determined to be out in the middle perfecting once more the late cut through third man for four that so many have mistaken for a fortuitous thick edge!

I really do need to get out more—especially onto the cricket field.

Phase Four

Moving On

53

What's Next

With the radiotherapy now complete it is starting to feel as though Miranda's battle with cancer is more behind us than in front of us. She now has just the six remaining Herceptin doses to complete; a two hour treatment once every three weeks through to Christmas. Prior to her diagnosis the thought of having to go to the hospital with such regularity would have seemed a real inconvenience but now it feels almost like a sense of freedom. It is amazing how events can change your perspective on matters. Of course there will still be the reconstruction to go at some point probably late next year and the six monthly check ups with the consultant. From a medical perspective she is not really "cured" of cancer for another four years and statistically the chances of it returning do not reduce to the level of the rest of us until 10 years have passed. But we have learnt to deal with the here and now and not try to project too far into the future.

Her body is now in recovery mode, her hair is growing back and the skin on her neck and front is starting to heal and look less sore and that is so good to see. All this means our thoughts are now turning to what next? Both Miranda and I have been so impressed, amazed and grateful for the support and work of all the nurses and the healthcare team that looked after her. The provision of Rachel, a Macmillan nurse specialist, to provide Miranda with support was a really valuable service and we have often been reassured by her when doubts occurred or we just needed some encouragement.

Having benefitted from such support we are keen to give something back, and Miranda and I have discussed over the past few weeks how we could do this. As you may be aware this month sees the Macmillan charity hold "The Worlds Biggest Coffee Morning" to help raise much needed funds. Always wanting to do things a little differently Miranda is in the process of organising an evening fundraising event instead. Calling it "Sugar and Spice—an Evening of Everything Nice", she has enlisted the support of local Suffolk food and drink producers including Paddy & Scotts coffee, Shawsgate Vineyard, James White juices, Hutton's Butchers, Leo's Deli and Suffolk Gold cheeses. She has also sold stand space to a few friends with small businesses. It promises to be a fun evening, although I will never know as it is girls only apparently, but I'm sure it will raise a few hundred pounds for Macmillan.

After what Miranda has been through, raising some funds to help provide other families affected by cancer with a "Rachel" feels a positive way to help us move forward and answer the "what's next?" question. Thanks for sticking with us.

54

New Look

Without doubt the highlight of this week has been Miranda's visit to the hairdresser on Thursday and the unveiling of her new look, wig free! She admitted on the morning to being more than a little apprehensive but, of course, she needn't have worried she looks absolutely stunning even if I'm a little biased. But honestly it's not just me that thinks that, judging by all the comments on her Facebook page. Apparently, the "elfin look" with short, slightly spiky hair, is so this year's "in" look don't you know!

Appearances are such funny things. We worry so much about how we look to others and we always are far harsher judges of our own appearance and style than virtually everyone else we meet. Why is that? Miranda, pre cancer, always had long, naturally blonde hair and without doubt the loss of her hair was one of the toughest things to come to terms with early on in her treatment. Her hair was part of what defined her and she felt like losing her hair was a little like losing her identity. And, to be honest, the loss of her breast presented similar challenges.

Bravely Miranda decided to have her hair cut short before the chemotherapy caused it to fall out. I think this proved to be a wise decision. Having experienced a naturally short hair look she gained the courage to go for a shorter wig than she might otherwise have done. And by having a short wig for almost eight months it feels less of a dramatic change to go for the natural "cropped" style now.

In fact Miranda would now admit that a short hair look has been strangely liberating. She would never have considered the thought of having her hair coloured or cut short but now that she has had no choice she will openly admit to looking forward to trying different styles that previously she would never have dared. What seemed such a horrible negative has turned into a real positive. Isn't that often the way with so many things in life?

For me the loss of the wig is tinged with a sadness that one gets at the loss of a faithful old friend. Obviously I hated watching Miranda having to suffer the side effects of chemo and seeing clumps of hair fall out as she tried to brush her hair was just horrible, but the wig has provided us with an opportunity to laugh at a time when such opportunities were few and far between. From the hilarious day spent choosing it in the first place in the wig shop that was like a step back in time, the wig has never been short of providing comedy moments. When the chemo was at its worst it was also a valuable barometer as to how Miranda was truly feeling. If the wig didn't go on in the morning you knew she was feeling really rubbish and that was bizarrely both helpful and reassuring for those of us around her at the time.

In the last few months, as I have explained before, Miranda has suffered from pre-menopausal hot flushes thanks to the ongoing effects of the chemotherapy. As her hair has grown back this has made the wearing of a wig on top of her hair when the flush strikes almost unbearable. No matter how many times I've seen it there is nothing funnier than watching her, in the middle of cooking tea or bathing the children, flinging her wig across the room to try to cool down. This sudden wig removal has also meant I have unearthed the wig in the most unusual of places. It has appeared under newspapers, on the cistern of the toilet, on the floor by the sofa, next to the cake tin etc. Each time there is the initial nanosecond shock of wondering what on earth I've uncovered, and then the smile of realisation. Of course now that she is no longer wearing it I feel duty bound to allow Miranda to enjoy such delights and have planned a few strategic places around the house where the wig may appear in the next few weeks! In the middle of a pile of ironing, for example, will be a great place—she won't find it for weeks!! Now promise me you won't let on to her will you. I'm so looking forward to Christmas as well—after the year we've had I can think of nothing better than her wig to replace the star on top of the tree as a one year only special!

One of the more unusual benefits of the wig is that it has allowed us to see which of our children really does most look like Miranda. I'm sure we are not the only family where this debate rages with various aunts and grandparents all claiming which child looks most like which parent. Rose and Millie have had great fun trying on Miranda's wig and glasses and we now have absolute proof as to who looks most like Miranda.

It is amazing how a hairstyle does transform your looks and we now have photographic evidence that it is actually Rose who takes after her Mum rather more than her sister. That debate is over for a while thanks to the wig.

55

The Wings to Fly

I was once told a story a few years ago that has resonated a little more with me over the last few months. You may be familiar with it, but it is the story of a naturalist who happens to find a chrysalis just as the butterfly is trying to break out of it. He watches enthralled for a while but it occurs to him just how much of a struggle it is for the butterfly to break out of its cocoon. The effort required seems almost painful and eventually the naturalist cannot bear watching the struggling butterfly anymore so, ever so gently, he peels away the skin of the chrysalis to allow the butterfly to break free. After a short while the butterfly's struggle is over and, thanks to the naturalist, it's free from the chrysalis. However the butterfly now has a new problem. It can't properly fly as its wings aren't strong enough. The butterfly needed the struggle and the pain of breaking out of the chrysalis to gain the strength to fly.

Clearly the moral of the story is that when we go through difficult times we can come through them a stronger person as a result. The last months have obviously given me the chance to evaluate whether this is true or not. And now that Miranda's through the worst of her treatment and her recovery is well under way, especially now the wig has been "retired," we've had the chance to reflect a little on what we've learnt from this journey with cancer. And if I'm honest, I'm not certain I'd describe myself as stronger for this experience. My perspective on life has been changed for certain, but stronger? Not so sure.

The other day I was challenged by someone who reminded me that, in the post I wrote on the day Miranda had her mastectomy, I'd suggested that one day I'd tackle a couple of posts about how my faith has been tested this year and also my thoughts on why God "allows" suffering, pain and bad things to happen. So in the odd quiet moment, or during the many road and train journeys of the last week or so, I've been wrestling with this question of why God allows us to go through painful experiences. And this is where I've got to so far . . . .

When Miranda was first diagnosed with breast cancer and we were trying to come to terms with what we were facing, a few people tried to reassure me that this was all part of God's big plan and that we might not understand it now but it would become clear in the future. I really struggle with that as an explanation. I mean, to accept this answer is to accept that God actually planned for my wife to go through this fear; planned for her to have treatment that causes all her hair to fall out; God intentionally allowed her to lose all the lymph nodes so that she has a lifetime of living with the threat of lymphodema; God has a plan for her to lose part of her femininity with the removal of her right breast; God planned for my wife to live with the very real fear that she may not get to see our children grow up; And yet He expects me to worship Him and pitch up every Sunday morning and sing about how great He is? Really? Actually if that is true, and I don't think it is, I don't want anything to do with such a God, no matter how good the "big plan" might be.

Then there is the "punishment" theory. A long while ago I really hurt and angered someone. They had every right to be hurt and be angry with me and, in their anger, they said that they didn't need to get angry and seek retribution, that God knew what had occurred and would deal with me. I found it quite a chilling statement at the time to be honest. So, was the close at hand witnessing of this terrible illness attacking my wife, a way of God punishing me for my previous actions? In my darkest moments the thought has crossed my mind but I've cast it out pretty quickly. Everything I have learnt about God is that He is all about grace and forgiveness so this kind of punishment doesn't even figure or make sense to me.

So having dismissed a "big plan" or punishment as the reason why God allows pain and suffering, I'm still no closer to explaining why He allows such events. Maybe the fact that these things happen is proof that God doesn't actually exist? I realise there are some of you who will find that the easiest and maybe the most obvious explanation. But for me, I can't believe that, as there have been many occasions over the last nine months when I have felt His presence so strongly.

I guess the best explanation I can come up with is that we live in a broken world. God gave us free will and we've chosen a way of living that He never intended and that's why He sent Jesus to show us how to live and to pay for our mistakes and, most importantly, to provide us with a hope of a better place to come. This world is broken but we have the hope that when we've journeyed through this life there is a place for us. A place where people don't fly planes into tall buildings, where wars don't happen, where giant waves don't sweep thousands of people to instant death, where thousands of helpless adults and children don't starve because it never rained and to a place where malignant lumps don't suddenly grow under your skin.

But the thing is, whilst I believe that to be true, I don't actually know that it is, for certain. And whilst I do cling to the hope that God provides, it wasn't easy to think of that when it's 2am and I'm walking down the empty, drab corridors of Ipswich Hospital with a wheelchair bound wife, who is being taken to the emergency admissions ward, sobbing in desperation at the thought of more time in hospital. And I'm walking and thinking that in 4 hours time I've got to explain to my two girls why their Mum who put them to bed isn't there when they wake up.

So here is what I think this journey with my wife's cancer battle has taught me. Life is not always about having the right answers, it is about having the right questions. You see I've had a long time to work out the whole "why does God allow us to suffer" question and I'm not sure I can answer it to my complete satisfaction. And actually I'm OK with that.

I think we are not intended to have all the answers to every question but we do need to think about the questions we ask.

What I've learnt is that I will never be able to explain why Miranda got breast cancer. I've said it before but of all the risk factors associated with breast cancer, the only one that Miranda has is that she is a woman. Why did she have to suffer this? How could this have happened? I don't have the answers to those questions, probably never will, but actually I now realise they are the wrong questions to ask. Even if I got a satisfactory answer to those questions it wouldn't change anything and I'm not sure I would feel any better for knowing.

The better question to ask having gone through this experience is what next? What do we do with what we've learnt and gone through? We could spend a lot of time looking back and wondering but we need to look forward and think what we can achieve, what we can make of the depth of experience we've been through.

And all of this brings me nicely back to my butterfly story. You see, as I mentioned before, I think the main point of that story is that we grow stronger through adversity. And maybe we do. But I look at that story now and I see it with a whole new perspective.

You see for any butterfly there will be a chrysalis experience. There will be a time of battle, of pain, of struggle, of uncertainty over the future, of doubt about whether it will ever get out of the chrysalis. But when it does, when it has broken out of the cocoon, it is faced with two options. It can either scratch around on a nearby leaf, living like it did before, as a caterpillar, whilst agonising over why it had to go through the difficulty and pain of the time in the chrysalis. Or, it can shake off the last few remnants of the chrysalis, look up and think, OK that experience is behind me, what's next?

And when it does that, it spreads its wings and experiences the wonder of flight for the very first time.

For me, just like the butterfly, what counts is not having the right answer, it is about asking the right question.

56

Any Steve, Graham or Harry

There are some weeks when the fact that Miranda is battling cancer can be conveniently tucked to the back of my mind and then there are others, like this week, when it seems an ever present thought rattling around my head.

I think there are a number of reasons for that this week. Firstly Miranda had her regular Herceptin treatment and also got a small lump which she has discovered in her neck checked out. Given the closeness of the lump to where her lymph nodes had been removed, and the fact that we now have an understandable aversion to lumps under her skin, this has been a slight worry. However the view is that it is unlikely to be anything sinister but next week's regular CT scan will go a little higher on her neck and they may do ultrasound too just to be on the safe side.

Miranda has also decided this week to go back to being a vegetarian, largely due to a nagging doubt about whether her decision to start eating meat two years ago may have led to her cancer. It has been something she had been considering for a while but her mind was made up after a conversation with a friend, a breast cancer survivor of some twelve years. This friend was told by her doctors that the two things which saved her life were the fact she was short and a vegetarian. It seems that there is a theory that breast cancer can feed off the growth promoters that are present in a lot of the meats that we eat. I've no idea why being vertically challenged helped by the way.

Of course I support Miranda's decision wholeheartedly even though this means I become a part time vegetarian too. There is no point us having separate meals and I can now look forward to having meat when we go out for dinner! I recognise that the debate over meat and its impact on cancer is ongoing and the research is largely inconclusive. But I think we have both found a certain degree of discomfort in the knowledge that after over twenty years of being a healthy vegetarian, Miranda was diagnosed with breast cancer just under a year after she started eating meat, despite attempting to only eat "happy" meat.

We will never know, I guess, why she got cancer but given the absence of other likely known risk factors, the closeness of her change of diet to the diagnosis is an unfortunate coincidence if nothing else.

But then again that is the randomness of cancer. You never know who it will hit and when. And this week there have been three high profile individuals who have lost their lives to cancer.

Steve Jobs was a visionary and someone who changed the way of the world. Through his Apple business he was the creator of Mac computers and the iPod, iPhone and iPad. He has been as revolutionary to the way we do business as Jethro Tull was to the farming industry and Henry Ford was to the transport industry. He was an individual that possessed the perfect storm of great business acumen, amazing vision and creativity with a wonderful eye for design and style.

Graham Dilley was a cricketing hero. He was the unsung batting partner to Ian Botham when they staged the most incredible comeback in Test Match history as England beat Australia and claim the Ashes in the early Eighties. One of the best opening bowlers of his generation he also became a highly respected coach once his playing days were over. At just 52 he passed away this week after a short battle with cancer.

And then there is Harry Moseley who, aged just 11, died last Saturday night. Many of you may not have heard of Harry but he is just as much of a hero as the other two guys. Over the last four years Harry has been battling brain cancer. Over the last two years he has run a campaign to raise funds for cancer research and doing all he can to help others benefit from improved treatment. Despite his age he has raised over £500,000 in those two years through various activities including getting people to buy bracelets and by doing public speaking. Yes that's right £500,000—half a million pounds. Makes my plans at fundraising seem almost pathetic by comparison.

I've never met Harry but I've been following him on Twitter, along with 83,000 other people, and via his website. He was an amazing boy. I may be over four times his age but over the last year he has taught me so much about dealing with cancer. He was an inspiration. His legacy will live on.

I'm realising that one of the ways that this cancer experience has changed me is the way that I view the deaths of high profile people to cancer. Of course, I was always sad, especially when, like this week, those who passed away were relatively young, but now it touches me in a way that is so much more raw and personal. I feel a connection to their families and a depth of sadness that to be honest still takes me by surprise. I guess it comes from the fact that I'm walking the walk their families have walked and when you learn of another tragic outcome, another life lost to cancer, it does hurt.

But that is the randomness of cancer. Irrespective of whether you run the second most profitable business in the world, or reached the very top in your favourite sport, or were just an 11 year old boy from Birmingham with an amazing passion for life and people, cancer can enter your world. And there is randomness about whether it will end your world or not too.

It is a respecter of no one—it can strike any Tom, Dick or Harry. Or as we learnt this week any Steve, Graham or Harry.

57

Start Spreading the News (Miranda's Fourth Blog Post)

Amazingly it has been six months since Miranda wrote her last post on this blog. So much has happened since then and with it being Breast Cancer Awareness month, it seemed an appropriate time for her to share a few thoughts. Here goes . . . .

So here we are. It's the middle of October. How did that happen? Where did the last 10 months go?

October brings many things.

It's the month when Autumn steps up a gear; the leaves are turning and falling; squirrels are superbusy; conker championships are in full flow; apples are at their best; and a celebration and thanksgiving for the harvest.

One member of our family particularly loves this month . . . Rose. It is her birthday this month you see; she says she loves October because the leaves change colour, but I think we could probably all guess the main reason for October being her favourite month! And it is always in this month that I ask myself why on earth I ever embarked on elaborate birthday cakes for my children, when a good old chocolate hedgehog (complete with Matchsticks for spines of course!) would have been perfectly adequate, or a cake in the shape of the number of the relevant age would have been equally ideal. But no! I set off at top speed, it would seem I tried to run before I could walk in the cake decorating department. And this year is no different . . . a Barbie cake! I'm already planning that next year will be a plain old number 7!

October also means many things to people in other countries. I took the opportunity to consult Wikipedia . . .

Did you know that it was the anniversary of the birth of Mahathma Ghandi on 2nd October? The same day was also International Day of Non-Violence—I wonder how many people failed to recognise this in their actions on that day?

In Germany they would have been celebrating Reunification of Germany in 1990 on 3rd October; now that was a momentous day in European history, and one which I actually remember!

And my big sister celebrated her birthday on 5th! (But naturally I couldn't possibly let on how many years she was celebrating!)

The month also celebrates numerous anniversaries of Independence in countries across the world, as well as National Days in Taiwan, Austria and Spain; Ochi Day (No Day) in Greece on 28th—I'm pondering how and why you celebrate a 'No Day'!—and of course Halloween on 31st.

October is also National Breast Cancer Awareness month. I expect you probably knew that already, with all the pink ribbons about at the moment. But it seemed an appropriate month for me to put my fingers to keys once more and blog this month.

According the Wikipedia, Breast Cancer Awareness is "an effort to raise awareness of breast cancer and reduce the disease's stigma by educating people about its symptoms and treatment options. Supporters hope that greater knowledge will lead to earlier detection of breast cancer, which is associated *with higher long-term survival rates, and that money raised for breast cancer will produce a reliable, permanent cure."*

It would seem a good time to acknowledge the good people of Bedfield. Earlier this month we joined together in the village sport's pavilion to enjoy a Harvest Lunch. Always great food and conversation, even if our girls did bring the average age down by a decade or two! But this is not a blog to tell of the ways of rural Suffolk, but to acknowledge the generosity of the village . . . with October being National Breast Cancer Awareness month the Women's Guild decided to donate all money to Breakthrough Breast Cancer. Every donation, no matter how small, might bring the researchers a step closer to achieving their goal.

If this blog achieves nothing else over this year, it is my absolute hope that it will succeed in raising awareness, from our own personal experience. Because if I am totally honest, I never thought breast cancer would happen to me. But it has, and if someone else can benefit from my experience, be encouraged to go and see their doctor to get an early diagnosis, or to try to keep going throughout the gruelling treatment, then that will make this whole exercise completely worthwhile.

I first visited my GP in January 2010; despite mammograms, biopsies and MRI, I was misdiagnosed for 10 months. Finally in November a mammogram showed some calcification, and another biopsy confirmed their concerns. This may sound really strange, but I was actually relieved that they had finally found something. So this led to a diagnosis, which was devastating of course, but a relief in a way to be able to get on with treatment.

I am not going back over this for any other reason than to highlight from my own personal experience the need to listen to and know your own body. We are the only ones that know our bodies well enough to notice slight changes. I wasn't happy to be told on one occasion that 'that is just how my breasts are', because I knew that they weren't! Every bit of me hopes that they can learn from my case, and that will subsequently ensure that a similar case is diagnosed sooner than mine. The Cancer Charities stress the benefit of early diagnosis, so whether it be changes in your breasts or any other part of your bodies, please do make an appointment to see your GP, and get that early diagnosis.

I know that it is still early days for me, but I can say for certain that it is possible to live through diagnosis and treatment and come out the other side, and still continue to live life as normally as possible throughout all of this. I think perspective and mindset is important, but this has all changed my outlook on cancer completely. I am no longer of the belief that cancer is always terminal, I feel I have a better understanding of what it means to have cancer, but—and there is a big BUT—I don't actually feel at the moment that I will ever be totally cured.

I remember reading an article on the BBC website a couple of months ago about a team of breast cancer researchers, whose aim is to find a means of treatment by which people learn to live with breast cancer; the aim that breast cancer will be treated like diabetes, with medication to keep it under control, but to never be cured from it.

I would be really happy with that. There is a small part of me that feels that this will not be the end to my experience with cancer, but I'm ok with that. I have experienced firsthand the wonders of modern medicine, and the care and wisdom of the doctors and nursing teams, and the diagnostic techniques and complex treatments that are available nowadays; and it is sobering to think that had this happened even just 10 years ago I may not be sitting here typing these thoughts and feeling as well as I do today.

And so my treatment continues. After this week's appointments, it is now looking likely that my Herceptin treatment may continue for another year. And not because of anything negative, just because it is possible that a longer course of Herceptin may prove beneficial to my long-term health—a medical conference in December will give the results of clinical trials, so I will know for certain after that if they consider it to be worth it or not. I think I'll take anything the NHS are willing to offer me!

So it appears that I have not reached the crossroads as soon as I had hoped, and so must continue on this road for a little while longer yet. Whilst I have been on this journey I have tried to look back and reflect a little upon the past 2 years. The one thing that is so clear to me is my responsibility to do all I can to support the campaign for awareness of this disease, be it through talking about it, blogging about it, or through fundraising. However I can I will be "spreading the news" although I think you'll be spared a further year of The Last Chocolate Brownie despite possible ongoing treatment (the blog will finish at Christmas) . . . after all I don't think our case for the last morsel of gooey chocolate cake is exactly authentic anymore! And despite my love of all things chocolate, I am actually rather grateful!

58

The Art of Elimination

One of the things that Miranda's cancer has robbed us off is the ability to have a proper holiday. We have been a little unlucky with timings as her radiotherapy fell during the summer school holidays and so we were unable to go away during that time and clearly the chemotherapy in the early part of the year meant life was too unpredictable to plan anything. So with this week being half term we have headed down to the New Forest and are having a week's holiday exactly a year since we had the last one! Boy am I ready for the break!

We travelled down last night and Miranda has once more chosen well and we are safely settled into a beautiful cottage on the edge of Lyndhurst. I've got a week planned of just enjoying time with the girls, all three of them, plus a bit of reading, some reflection and a little bit of writing—I need to turn this blog into a book and so I plan to edit previous posts over the course of the week. So many of the everyday tasks can be forgotten and I think it will be a great week!

On the health front it is great to see that Miranda is able to join in with all activities such as running around with the girls. She is starting to look really well again, the radiotherapy skin burn has gone, she has loads more energy and the sparkle is back in her eyes. It's true that her nails are still a bit damaged from the chemo and her hair, although growing, is still shorter than she would like, but that is all pretty minor in the scheme of things. Her latest hospital visits have gone well; there is talk of continuing the Herceptin treatment for another year, just to reduce further the chances of the cancer returning. The lump in her neck will have some ultrasound but seemed to cause little concern to the medics and although the latest CT scan showed a small area of shadowing on her lungs this is thought to be due to damage from the radiotherapy and not anything sinister. They will monitor again in January.

My reading list for the week includes Don Miller, Trevor Waldock, Howard Shultz (Starbucks CEO) and Rob Bell; all of them would feature in my favourite authors list. I'm reading again Rob Bell's "Drops Like Stars" which has inspired previous posts in this blog. In it he talks about the art of elimination—the fact that sometimes it is not all about what we can add to improve things, quite often we need to work out what we need to eliminate to create something better. Bell gives the great analogy of the most wonderful statue which has been created out of stone. What makes the statue so beautiful is what the sculptor took away, not what he added. In every basic block of stone is an incredible statue waiting to be created. I think that is such a clever analogy but a year ago, when I first read the book, I didn't fully appreciate the point quite like I do now. When you discover your wife is battling cancer you gain a certain focus and clarity about stuff that you never had before.

When Miranda's diagnosis came along I didn't find myself thinking about what work I wanted doing on the house, or getting our rather outdated TV replaced, or what other responsibilities or roles I could secure for myself. Suddenly life was all about how I could support her and our daughters best, how I could ensure we spent more time together. All the unnecessary and trivial stuff in my life was ditched. But the challenge to eliminating stuff is that it is counter-cultural to the world in which we live.

I was reminded of this fact in a simple way as I stood in line at Costa Coffee this morning. The barista was trying to encourage everyone to add to their coffee order—an extra shot, a syrup, chocolate on top, a pastry to go with it. I don't blame her she was just doing her job trying to upsell, and doing it pretty well, but it reminded me of the art of elimination. I mean if you love coffee, you just want a coffee, perfectly brewed, well made, nothing added don't you? Why should the addition of other things make the coffee any better?

And it occurred to me that we treat life just like Costa do coffee too. Just about every marketing message we hear is trying to convince us that life would be better if we added more stuff and I think it is dawning on me that this probably isn't true. In the past I've spent far too much time worrying about what I want but don't have, planning how I can add more to my life, be it a new flat screen TV, or a new role or project I can take on. Over the last year I've realised that the real skill, and more importantly the real benefit, comes from working out what we can eliminate from our lives. What can we actually take away from our activities and our desires that will actually enhance our life? I'm not for one moment trying to suggest that owning a flat screen TV is wrong by the way but it is amazing what a life threatening disease to your wife does to put those kinds of desires into a metaphorical "box" marked trivial.

So, as we hopefully come out the other side of Miranda's cancer battle, I'm trying really hard to maintain that focus on taking away rather than adding to. I want to practice the art of elimination. Just like the sculptor I'm hoping to chip away until I reveal something quite beautiful. That has got to be worth the effort don't you think?

59

Looking Up to the Stars

Today I'm experiencing that "end of the holiday" mindset where I am trying to get back to normality and thoughts of work and all the regular stuff that life is full of. From tomorrow, gone will be the gentle start to the morning, lazy breakfast and taking the day as it comes. It will all be about early starts, meetings and deadlines.

We have had a lovely week off and spending time together has been great. Ask the girls what their favourite part of the holiday was and they would probably say it was the visit to Peppa Pig World or the day trip on the ferry to the Isle of Wight. They've never been on a ferry before so that naturally was full of excitement and Peppa Pig World was just as you'd expect a theme park to be! There were lots of rides which even Millie was able to go on—I was very pleased that she was too small to go on George's dinosaur ride on her own and needed me to accompany her! And none of the rides were too scary for either of the children, or either of their parents come to that! Peppa Pig World also helped teach us the value of patience, it was half term after all, and the average wait for a ride was about 25 minutes! The stars of the show were, of course, Peppa and George themselves and Millie was so pleased to get a chance to meet them and hold their hands. Her wide eyed excitement was just a joy to witness.

For me the favourite holiday memory was our walk in the New Forest. I think there is something special about the chance to just soak in the beauty of our surroundings when there is no time pressure or real purpose to the walk. We simply wandered through the forest following a path without knowing where it would lead us. We encountered the occasional pony who seemed to be appreciating the environment as much as we were. There was an incredible richness to the colours of the leaves on the trees, from the shades of browns to the fiery reds and ambers that adds warmth to the autumn hue of the forest. There was crispness and freshness to the air of the kind that seems to seep into you in the most invigorating of ways. Miranda was busy identifying the variety of birdsongs that provided the soundtrack to our walk while Rose was "treasure hunting" for various items for her scrapbook. Amongst her best finds were a butterfly wing and a discarded horse's hoof. Millie loved splashing in all the puddles until the cracks in her wellies failed and her feet became soaked requiring me to carry her for the rest of the walk.

We walked until we found a stream gently meandering through this copse and wondered why the water took such a curvy route and then we headed back to the car. As we left the copse it started to rain quite heavily and I pulled Millie's hood over her head, held her close to me to keep her dry as best I could, and we marched on. Every few paces I was encouraged by this little voice from beneath the hood saying "thank you Daddy, I'm not getting wet." After a while Millie went quiet and as I gently lifted her hood I realised she had fallen asleep. I treasured the moment and despite the rain and the weight of my daughter I didn't want the walk to end. We arrived back at the car quicker than I expected.

The afternoon was one more reminder of how we are surrounded by the beauty of nature and that I don't take enough time out to create moments to appreciate it. How do I let that happen? I guess it is so often the fast paced life we live that means we forget those things we should be grateful for.

Like our health for example.

Whilst Miranda is feeling loads better compared to earlier in the year she still has the remnants of the chemotherapy in her system and the thoughts of reconstructive surgery to come. Her shoulder, where the lymph nodes were removed, regularly aches and she is accepting that this is now probably how it will always be. I think she is also experiencing the inevitable concerns that any cancer victim encounters at this stage in their recovery. Suddenly the everyday tweaks and twinges that we all get from time to time raise the nagging doubt of whether they are actually the start of something more sinister. And those concerns are hard to dispel.

We both know that we must look forward, that we must remain positive, but there are days when that is easier said than done. Bizarre as it might sound but when she was dealing with the chemo and the radiotherapy it was almost easier to do this. The treatment she was going through provided a clear reference point and the goal was to get through it. And she did, brilliantly in fact. Now of course the goal is a little fuzzier and so it can be hard work to look forward and ignore the odd symptom she experiences which might be a sign of the cancer returning.

Never again will I take for granted the fact that I wake up every morning free from concerns about my health.

And tonight as I put Rose to bed we looked out of her bedroom window. Thanks to the putting the clocks back last night she now goes to bed when it is completely dark.

We gazed up at the stars in the sky, grateful for the fact that we live in the depth of the countryside and our view is not spoiled by light pollution, noting just how brightly they shine.

"Isn't it amazing Daddy that we get this star show every night," Rose said in a simplistically, profound way that only a small child can.

But it got me thinking. Imagine if the stars in the sky could only be seen once a year. What an event it would be. People would camp out all night, hold star gazing parties, it would be covered by the media and we would all feel desperately cheated if it was a really cloudy night and we had to wait another year before we got a proper view.

So does the fact that the stars are out every night make them any less amazing a sight? And when was the last time that you took five minutes to just enjoy the night sky? I always feel so dwarfed by the sheer scale of what I see, knowing that some of the stars I'm looking at actually burnt out years ago but as they are hundreds of light years away they only appear to us now. Incredible.

For all of us there will be times when life is really tough and because of that I'm grateful that this week has taught me, once more, that we need to make sure that every so often we get our head up and look to the stars.

There is so much to be thankful for.

60

If the Cup Fits . . . .

Last week when I put Millie to bed I was explaining to her that our holiday was over and that everything would be back to normal. I went on to mention that this meant that I had to go back to work and Rose, her sister, would have to go back to school.

"Yes Daddy, I know," she said adding "and Mummy will have to go back to the hospital"

Millie is 3 and it made me realise that for her, "normal" is Dad at work, sister at school and Mum having to regularly go to the hospital. That is what we do, or at least that is what it seems like for virtually the last year. And to a certain extent Millie's perspective is not far from the truth, Miranda has indeed been back to the hospital again this week. This time it was for her regular dose of Herceptin but she was also able to get an unscheduled meeting with her McMillan Nurse Specialist and Oncologist. They were able to provide some very welcome reassurance about the symptoms Miranda has been experiencing over the last few weeks. They were able to confirm that these symptoms are perfectly normal, only what is to be expected after all that Miranda has been through, and they are not concerned that they could be any indication that her cancer is returning. That was a really helpful meeting to have.

The other meeting that Miranda had was with the prosthetics clinic. The purpose of this was to provide

Miranda with a more permanent prosthetic breast now that her skin has recovered from the radiotherapy. This will be what she will use until she has reconstructive surgery late next year. As those of you who follow Miranda on Facebook will already know, I wasn't allowed to attend this meeting. Apparently my uncontrolled sniggering at the last meeting when artificial breasts and, wait for it, support groups (childish I know but still funny) were discussed, meant that Miranda felt it was best she attended this particular meeting on her own.

Clearly I was gutted. I mean it transpired that the prosthetics clinic is held in a room which is floor to ceiling mirrored cupboards, full of boxes of breasts. Can you imagine?! I also felt I could have constructively added to the debate about which breast was the best fit, you know, held it in my hand that type of thing. No?! OK maybe it was best I didn't go!

Until now Miranda has had a "comfy." This is basically a cushioned pad which is inserted into a pocket on a specially adapted bra. The problem with this is that it doesn't move as her body moves. The result is that Miranda occasionally has to make the odd discreet adjustment to get everything back in the right place. Think of Cissie and Ada, the older women characters played by the late Les Dawson and Roy Barraclough and you've got the picture!

Up until now the only experience we have had of a prosthetic breast is the one that Miranda has for swimming, which clearly is designed to get wet. When not in use this lives in a box in Miranda's sports bag, although there has been the odd occasional hilarious moment when Millie has got hold of it and paraded around the room with the breast balanced delicately on her head. Feel free to add your own punchline here! I must admit, with Millie being a non swimmer, I always felt reassured by this addition to our swimming equipment. I mean, if ever Millie's armbands failed, Miranda can just whip out the implant and Millie could safely get herself to the edge with this improvised "floatation" aid.

Anyway I digress. The key point is that Miranda is making one more step forward in her recovery from this whole process and will have a more permanent solution to her mastectomy. From her perspective, the key thing is that she will soon be able to go back to wearing more normal bras and tops and that will feel like a real step forward.

I realise that for many women the loss of a breast is a major psychological blow and I can completely understand why that would be so. I can also imagine that for some people, the light hearted approach we have taken to this subject will seem both inappropriate and maybe even disrespectful. Clearly this is not our intention and I apologise if you feel this is the case. Simply put, this is our story about how we have tried to deal with Miranda's cancer and all its side effects. I am amazed at how well Miranda has coped with the physical changes she has experienced and, to be brutally honest, the physical things such as the wig and the false breast have been a welcome source of humour for us in what has been a pretty dark time. I am so grateful that I have a wife who is able to deal with these matters in such a positive and humourous way as I find laughter to be the best way for me to deal with such situations too. I hope you will understand.

Of course I am all too aware that in time the loss of a breast is something that Miranda may find more difficult to deal with but for now she is looking forward to the practical benefits of going back to her wardrobe and having a greater choice of outfits. After all if the cup fits . . . .

61

We All Make Mistakes

Well we all make mistakes . . . . as the Dalek said climbing off the dustbin!

Sorry that is a really old school joke that I'm afraid I couldn't resist repeating once I'd decided on the title. I appreciate it will obviously only be funny to those of you who were Dr Who fans during the late '70's but it's not worthy of any further explanation trust me.

But the point is we all do don't we? Make mistakes I mean. You see earlier this year I made one at work. As mistakes go this was a big, fat, ugly one. A mistake that had a £ sign in front of it and a fair few "0's" after it. I could have made all sorts of excuses but the harsh, honest reality is that a couple of years ago I didn't read something as closely as I should and just signed it off. The reality of my mistake came to light earlier this year. Nightmare! Obviously I felt really bad about this, but the biggest learning curve in all this came from the reaction of my fellow Directors. The grace and support they showed me was unequivocal and there was a sense of let's just move on, we are all in this together. Now, let's be clear, I wouldn't say they could be described as happy about the situation and we've made some changes going forward. I don't sign those sorts of documents now without someone else checking them, which I actually think is a very good idea to be honest. And guess what, by showing me their support in such a situation, my fellow Directors have guaranteed I'm doing all I can to make up for my mistake and actually it's now looking that it might not be quite as expensive an error as first feared.

So what's the point of this confession you may wonder? Well now that we have had a moment or two to reflect on all that has happened over the past year, Miranda and I have been considering how we deal with her misdiagnosis. By way of a reminder, Miranda had been to see the Breast Consultant twice during the year before they found her cancer. She had mammograms, biopsies, ultrasound and MRI scans which all missed it. Indeed on the second visit the Consultant famously told her that "the lump was just how her breasts are".

When I retell this story many people have said something along the lines of "surely you are going to sue them."

And I understand why they say that. It is part of the culture that we live in which means we are actively encouraged to sue if anything we have bought or any event has happened to us and has been negative. We don't have "accidents" any more—an "accident" has to have been someone's fault and we should make them pay for it. Literally. The country is now covered with "ambulance chasing", no-win-no-fee lawyers looking to make some money out of someone's misfortune.

I'm not going to pretend the thought about making a claim hasn't crossed my mind. I think we would have a pretty good chance of winning too. But when I analyse it, I find myself wondering what the purpose of such action would be. I mean do I think that Miranda's Consultant wilfully or maliciously misdiagnosed Miranda's lump? Absolutely not. I saw the look in her face when she had to break the news to us that the lump was in fact cancerous and it had now spread into her lymph nodes. She knew she'd made a mistake and I know how she felt because I've made mistakes too. Haven't we all? Just because she does the job that she does shouldn't mean those mistakes carry a far higher price than they do for those of us in less life critical job roles. I'm so grateful I don't get sued every time I make a mistake! Imagine the atmosphere at work if we all worked in that kind of environment.

To be honest, I struggle with the whole concept of suing someone after a mistake or an accident. Clearly if someone caused you pain or suffering deliberately and in a negligent way then I understand the need to provide some kind of recompense. I also understand that if the mistake leads to the desperate situation where the person is left needing long term care, or with life changing injuries, then they are absolutely entitled to all the money they need to live out their life in the best way they can. But when it is a genuine misdiagnosis then why do we seek money from them? By accepting a cash payment we are putting a value on the "loss" we have experienced.

Take Miranda's case, if we sued the Consultant we would effectively be saying that all she has gone through over the last year, the loss of her breast, the chemo, the side effects, could be "put right" by the payment of a few thousand pounds. How do you put a value on that? I do think it is impossible to put a value on my wife's breast—it is actually priceless! (I do take a silly amount of satisfaction to have worked that last statement into my post by the way!).

I defy anyone to try to justify a payment that adequately compensates us for going through what Miranda has suffered over the last 10 months, or what else she may face in the future. So why should we try to sue for an amount? Whatever we got financially would seem so irrelevant.

And my other consideration is that any money we got would indirectly affect the treatment available to others. I think sometimes people forget that liability payments do have an origin. Indirectly they will filter back to the NHS budget and that means less money to pay for the drugs that have helped rid Miranda of the cancer in her body. We genuinely would rather leave it in the NHS. Surely that is putting it to far better use?

Moreover, by suing are we likely to help ensure that less misdiagnosis happens in the future? I very much doubt it. Miranda is relatively young to have breast cancer, it is much more difficult to diagnose in younger people as the tissue is that much denser. This was a simple, honest mistake and whether we sue will make no difference at all to the likelihood of another mistake being made.

Miranda has been back to hospital twice this week, to visit the Consultant and to have her MUGA scan to check her heart. Just to clarify the Consultant Miranda now sees is not the same one who misdiagnosed the cancer initially. We would have stayed with the original Consultant but for her taking annual leave just as Miranda was due for her mastectomy. The second and current Consultant has been brilliant in every regard. All this week's news is good! The mammogram on her remaining breast was clear, the Consultant was impressed about how well Miranda's scar is healing and there was more discussion about the options on reconstruction which will probably happen at the end of 2012. The lump on her neck was given some ultrasound investigation and there are no concerns that it is anything suspicious. All just as we could have hoped and very, very encouraging.

So let's just hope they are not missing anything this time around!

I realise that we may be in a minority by taking this approach to the misdiagnosis, but sometimes I think we can all learn so much by taking a step back and asking why we are "following the crowd" in the actions we take. Some of you may think that we are mistaken and are wrong to not pursue what is our "entitlement". And you may well be absolutely right. But I suppose it does us all good to live a little counter-culturally from time to time.

So all those cold calling, no win, no fee, legal firms needn't start phoning us. We won't be trying to sue Miranda's first Breast Consultant and why should we? After all, we all make mistakes sometimes don't we?

62

Big Boys Don't Cry

It's fair to say that most of the posts in this blog have been written "in the moment". By that I mean I get a thought, or something has happened in Miranda's cancer battle, and I have written the post in response and posted it straight away. There has been the occasional post that I've written and then felt I wanted to reflect on it a little before posting. And there are one or two posts that I've written and which for various reasons have remained in my draft file. I wrote the first part of this post back in January and I'm rather ashamed to admit that I was probably a little too proud to publish it at the time. It has just sat there and now I've finally plucked up the courage to hit the "publish" button.

You see I was bought up in an era when I was always told not to cry. Even when I was as young as my children are now, I remember being told to stop crying—"big boys don't cry" was the usual comment thrown at me when the tears were falling down my cheeks. Being a bloke too has meant I have always tried to suppress any emotion escaping, stiff upper lip and all that. Any crying I've done as an adult, has to a large extent been done in private with no one else around.

So when Miranda was diagnosed with cancer I felt an enormous pressure, self induced I hasten to add, to be strong for her. In reality I think over the first month it was actually the other way around! Miranda was incredibly strong and whilst she naturally had the odd tearful moment these were fairly few and far between. For me I just about managed to stay strong when I was with her, but when I was on my own I was in bits. I developed an art of working out where and when to have a good cry without embarrassing myself too much!

For example, 48 hours after Miranda was diagnosed I had my annual Christmas meal with the head office team at work. Having had the day in the office I knew I wouldn't get through the evening without crying so I took myself off to the health club and cried my eyes out in the shower. Its pretty easy to cover up crying when you are in the shower! I learnt too that you can cry when driving. I just had to make sure I allowed sufficient time before I got to the meeting for the red eyes to go. Oh and its not great to cry if you are likely to get stuck in traffic! Or whilst queuing at traffic lights; that can get embarrassing!

I've also shed the odd tear or two with Rose when Miranda was having a tough time with the chemo. Often this was brought on by something Rose had said which just broke my heart but, having now had time to reflect I think crying with her was a good thing to do. It legitimised for Rose that it was OK to cry and enabled me to explain to her that crying is a natural way of the body responding when we sad just like we laugh when we find something funny.

That's the lesson I have learnt over the last year. There is obviously a time to be strong for your family but that must be balanced with the need to recognise that crying is a natural human response to a situation we find upsetting and, male or female, child or adult, it is OK to let our emotions be released through the act of crying.

And I was reminded of this post yesterday as I watched Shay Given visibly crying live on TV over the death of his close friend Gary Speed prior to kick off in the match between Swansea and Aston Villa. Later Robbie Savage was also seen on TV visibly upset whilst paying tribute to Speed. Clearly big boys do cry.

I've written about this before but since Miranda has been diagnosed with cancer I have found the death of high profile individuals much more difficult to deal with than I had before. And Gary Speed's tragic death in the most awful of circumstances was no different. It rocked me and I could think of little else throughout the day. I think the reason for this is that the experience of Miranda battling potentially life threatening illness brings inevitable thoughts of losing the person closest to you. And that's a scary, frightening thought. And so when someone you "know" passes away there is a sharpness and rawness to the emotions that get evoked.

I can only begin to imagine what Gary Speed's family are going through right now but there must be a sense of total disbelief and the burning question of why did someone they love so much feel they had no option but to take their own life. One of the deepest parts of the tragedy of a suicide is that the question of why is one to which there is seldom ever an answer.

Less than 48 hours after Gary Speed's death is clearly far too early for any explanation as to why he committed suicide but there is clearly much media speculation that he was suffering from depression which he kept well hidden from his public persona. Incredibly well hidden it seems to those of us who saw him appear on TV just hours before he took his own life.

I have had first hand experience of depression hitting a member of my immediate family. It is clearly an illness and not a state of mind or approach to life which so many people can so easily mistake it for. In many cases it is a chemical imbalance that effects the mind and in the case of my own family once the correct dose of tablets was discovered to balance out these chemicals, the transformation in behaviour was both incredible and unrecognisable from the depressed state they had previously been in.

The biggest problem with mental illness is that it is an unseen killer. According to NHS statistics just under 20 people a day take their own lives in the UK. Over the past day I've been thinking a bit about our attitude towards depression. As a result of Gary Speed's death there has been a lot of debate on Twitter and in the press about it. Unlike the lumps under your skin that arrive with cancer there are no obvious outward signs of depression and therefore people understand much less about it. It has made me wonder whether the reaction to this blog would be different if it was about my wife's battle with depression rather than with cancer. I'm not sure.

Prior to experiencing depression within my family I would definitely have subscribed to the "just pull yourself together" school of thought. Now I realise that "pulling yourself together" is precisely what someone with depression just cannot do no matter how much they may want to or try to. You can no more "pull yourself together" to get over depression than you can "pull yourself together" to get over cancer. And I so wish more people realised this.

So many people get angry with the person who has taken their own life and question how they could hurt those so close to them. It is an understandable reaction but the evilness of depression is that at the point of taking their own life, the individual's mind is so unbalanced that they genuinely don't think they will be causing any hurt or creating so much pain. It is a truly tragic illness in every respect.

If depression turns out to be the cause Gary Speed's death, my only hope is that some good can come out of it and that mental illness becomes something that is more openly discussed and understood as a result of the media attention his passing generates.

And once more I'm left realising that the situation we have faced over the last twelve months is just a walk in the park compared to the challenges other people face.

I might be a big boy and I might cry from time to time but I have so much to be thankful for too.

63

A Big Hairy Audacious One

So the build up to Christmas is well and truly under way in the Courteen household. Last weekend we went back to Miranda's parents for the traditional orchestra weekend. Miranda and her Mum both play in the Stratford-Upon-Avon Symphony Orchestra while her Dad is the conductor. The Christmas concert this year included the Nutcracker Suite so both our two girls were allowed to attend. It made for a very late night for both of them but it has become part of our family Christmas tradition. I also make full use of the fact that with rehearsals taking place on the Sunday afternoon I get to do some Christmas shopping with my two girls.

This weekend we've been to Lou and Julians, Miranda's sister and brother-in-law. We've had a great time, exchanged presents and just chilled out. Our two nieces get on so well with our two daughters so it has been a really relaxing time. And now we are home and Miranda is decorating the tree, Harry Connick Junior is blasting out the Christmas songs on the CD and I'm writing this post. It feels like a normal Christmas. That is a good thing.

Miranda has had a whole week without any hospital visits. That is still a rarity and so it is something she has really enjoyed. Next week is her Herceptin week and she hopes to hear whether they are going to continue with this treatment for another year or not. We are really trying to look forward rather than back. With the anniversary of

Miranda's diagnosis looming large and the start of a new year just around the corner, we want to see this as a real watershed opportunity to "move on".

Miranda is going to write one final reflective post and I have a couple of other posts that I want to write before I will put up the final post on Christmas Eve. That will be precisely a year to the day since this blog began. We both really think that our turn to claim the last chocolate brownie is over and maybe it is time to "pass the plate of brownies" on to others. Of course it doesn't mean that our story is complete, just that we need to change the context in which we tell it. With that in mind I have set up a new blog which will be starting in January. Reflecting the fact that we live in Suffolk which is renowned for it's flat terrain and expansive skies with incredible sunsets the blog will be called "Under Beautiful Skies".

The other way in which we intend to make this move forward and to move on from the "living with cancer" experience is to give ourselves a goal to focus on for next year.

And if you are going to set yourselves a goal then I think it might as well be a big, hairy audacious one otherwise what is the point frankly!

With that in mind we have set ourselves the challenge of raising £20,012 in 2012 with the proceeds split between Breakthrough Breast Cancer and the Woolverstone Wish campaign.

We have chosen these two charities as the beneficiaries of our fundraising for fairly fundamental and obvious reasons. The Woolverstone Wish is a campaign to raise much needed funds to help improve the quality of facilities on offer to those people receiving care in the Oncology Day Unit at Ipswich Hospital. Miranda has spent a lot of time here over the past year and has experienced first hand the incredible work the staff team carry out with limited resources. It seems pretty natural that we would like to do something to reflect our gratitude for the work they do whilst, at the same time, help others who are going through the horrendous experience Miranda has been through, to do so with a little more comfort.

There has been much made in the press over the last week about how people can avoid cancer by changing their lifestyle. There have been figures quoted of around 40% of all cancers being attributable to the lifestyle choices people make. For Miranda, her cancer clearly was in the 60% for which there is no obvious link to any lifestyle causes. Breakthrough Breast Cancer are working hard to research the causes of this horrible disease with the ultimate aim of finding a way to beat it. We both think this is a great aim, a big, hairy, audacious goal in its own right and one that we want to support as best as we can.

So there we are. A few weeks ago I wrote about the fact that we needed to ask ourselves the right questions and accept that we didn't have all the answers. We are learning to accept that we will never know why Miranda has had to go through this horrible cancer experience and we realise that we need to stop asking why and start asking what next instead.

So the answer to what's next is partly that we are going to take on a big, hairy and audacious goal.

It feels like a massive challenge but, funnily enough, just about this time last year we took on a challenge that also seemed massive and big and hairy and scary too. At least this new one is self imposed and I really like that!

64

What's In A Date?

Isn't it strange the emotions that we can attach to dates? Obviously we love to celebrate birthdays and certain dates hold special significance for us. My Mum, for example, always wants to mark August 19th as it is the date that she lost both her Dad and her husband. They passed away 37 years apart but it seems incredible that the anniversary of their deaths' fall on the same day. Whilst my Mum's desire is perfectly understandable, I prefer to remember my Dad on his birthday and on Father's Day rather than remembering the day he died.

And certain events link dates too. I will remember forever that my youngest niece was born on the same day that England, led by Michael Vaughan, finally recaptured the Ashes from the Aussies. The challenge is to remember the actual date that these two events happened! Only joking Sophie; I know it is September 12th really!

So all of that preamble is a way of leading up to saying that today is a date that is memorable for all the wrong reasons. Today marks the one year anniversary of Miranda's diagnosis of breast cancer. It was on this day last year that we learnt that our world was about to be turned upside down. And much as I try to dismiss it, I can't help but have that thought and the emotion of that day at the forefront of my mind this morning. In a slightly ironic way, Miranda is marking the anniversary with a trip to the hospital and her

Dave Courteen

regular dose of Herceptin. That kind of sums up her year really!

But, strange as it may seem, as I look back on all that we have been through, I think that the overriding feeling I have is of being thankful:

I'm thankful for how well Miranda now looks;

I'm thankful that our children have seemingly coped so well with the situation;

I'm thankful that the cancer has gone;

I'm thankful for the incredible support and love we have received from friends and family throughout the year;

I'm thankful for all the things that this experience has taught me;

and I'm thankful for all that we can now look forward to.

I can't pretend that the last year has been the best ever and I can't pretend that today doesn't invoke the odd feeling of sadness but I want to leave you with this thought. Not long after Miranda's diagnosis I was feeling especially down and was heading off to a meeting for work. I checked my Twitter feed and found a link to the following verse. With delicious timing it really lifted my spirits so I thought I'd share it with you:

What Cancer Cannot Do

Cancer is so limited that:
It cannot cripple love
It cannot shatter hope
It cannot corrode faith
It cannot kill friendship
It cannot suppress memories
It cannot silence courage

262

It cannot invade the soul
It cannot steal eternal life
It cannot conquer the spirit

There are indeed many things that cancer cannot do. I hope that by including that verse here there may be just one person reading this that will be as equally encouraged and helped as I was a year ago.

At the time I first read it, I wanted to believe it, I wanted to know that it was true.

One year on I can report, irrespective of the date, it is true.

65

Mastectomy—A Girl's Perspective

Being someone who likes a little neatness and order (you should see my CD collection!) we have just a week left of "The Last Chocolate Brownie"! I am determined that the blog will conclude on Christmas Eve exactly one year after it started. So this weekend Miranda is making her final post and will reflect on what she has learnt from the last year of living with cancer, and a mastectomy. We thought it would be good to close with a kind of "his and hers" review of what we have experienced. Miranda is going first and I will share my thoughts later this week before the final post goes up on Christmas Eve. So now that you know the plan here are the thoughts of my very brave wife . . . .

As I sit and ponder over this, my final contribution to the blog, I can't help but find myself considering and reflecting a little on the last 12 months. You could say it's been a funny old year, and it feels quite surreal to think back on it now. This time last year we were all battling ice and snow; I would regularly wonder whether Dave would actually make it to work or more importantly whether he would actually make it home again. For the first time that I remember, Dave conceded that my ever-cautious Dad may actually have a point, and that it would probably pay to be sensible and keep a shovel and warm clothes in the car . . . just in case! A sure sign it was a hard winter!

When I think back over the course of events, and what felt like endless appointments over that previous year (and of course this last one), the day that remains with me vividly is, not surprisingly, the day I was diagnosed. When I was given the diagnosis, whilst shocking and devastating, it was somehow deep down what I expected. And yet I can't recall that meeting quite as well as the rollercoaster of emotions I was feeling during the subsequent 3 hours when I was left alone to mull over what I had been told whilst I awaited my surgery slot to have the lymph node in my neck removed. I don't think the nurses in that department quite knew what to do with this tearful woman, because of course they had no idea about what I had just been told by the Breast Consultant. Inter-departmental communication can be at times a little lacking!

But that really does seem such a long time ago and now life has returned pretty much to normal.

And it was 'normal' that I have tried so desperately hard to cling on to over the past 12 months and in a number of ways feel I have managed it:

My wig (which for an NHS hairpiece I don't think was too bad!) enabled me to carry on life as normal to the outside world—obviously I had my 'hoodie days' in the privacy of my own home, but if someone passed me in the street, I would like to think they would not have known what treatment I was going through;

During the months of chemo, my mum would ask me how I was in a morning, and I would say "I'm ok", naturally she was sceptical because apparently I would "always say that!", but if I was up, showered, dressed, and ready to take Rose to school, I was, in my book, "ok";

In my mind I had to remain visible to the world, because I knew that if I shut myself away then family life would change to beyond what our girls would recognise as normal and I would assume the "patient role" (as my sister Lou, a trained nurse described it) which I was determined not to do!;

And as far as the outside world is concerned I continue to look like the next woman, albeit one with short hair and who no longer flashes her cleavage!

The hair I can just about cope with, and although it is not yet long enough to have a hairstyle of choice it continues to grow steadily—3ʳᵈ trip to the hairdressers in 4 months next week incidentally, I had never realised quite how expensive, time-consuming and cold it is to have short hair! However the lack of cleavage is harder to accept.

If you are long-term followers of this blog, you may recall the decision-making I went through when deciding on what type of reconstruction to opt for . . . and then the immense disappointment when that decision was taken away from me because my blood results were too low and the risk of infection subsequently too high, ultimately meaning that I was unable to have immediate reconstruction.

My decision to have immediate reconstruction was so that I would wake up from the operation as complete as when I went to sleep. I believed that that was fundamental to my ability to cope with the psychological and physiological effects of the surgery. And when that decision was taken away from me, I felt awash with panic and dread at the thought of having to remain "incomplete" for at least 15 months and having to face further surgery next year.

The prospect of seeing my scar for the first time also filled me with dread, but all I can say is that the thought of it was so much worse that the reality. Isn't that so often the case? We build something up in our head to something much bigger than it actually is, and when we are faced with it, we acknowledge, accept and adjust. Because there is really nothing else we can do.

So I have come to terms with how I am for the short term. It looks a bit odd, but then other than my husband and children, no one else sees that. Everyone else sees "normal". It is much less drastic and life-changing surgery than might occur for other types of cancer, so for that I have to be incredibly grateful. And I have the opportunity at a later date to have that abnormality rectified. What is really strange, and has surprised me enormously, is that I don't actually miss my other breast—just glad to be rid of it if I'm honest—and I didn't grieve the loss that I've heard is very normal in this situation. But I miss having a cleavage. Not that I overtly flaunted it, but it limits what I wear, makes me feel a bit less than whole and that I've lost a bit of my femininity. I realise that is such a small price to pay, and probably touches on the side of vanity if my biggest issues are just aesthetic.

I have come to realise throughout this whole process that how you look does actually have a strong correlation to how you feel. I have come across a cancer support charity called Look Good . . . Feel Better, via a blog I have been following recently, written by the Beauty Editor of LOOK magazine, Sophie Beresiner, who was also diagnosed with breast cancer last December and whose journey has pretty much mirrored my own. Both Sophie's blog and the philosophies of the charity have reassured my need to look "normal" to the outside world.

How often do we wear a public face? And some of us get very good at wearing it. I have worn my public face quite often over the past 12 months, but because I managed to convince myself that I felt OK it became easier to convince others I was doing OK. Equally, if someone had told me just over 12 months ago that I would be able to feel confident with short hair and only one breast I don't think I would actually have believed them. But amazingly I've discovered I can. How? Because it's not vain to be concerned about our appearance—if we feel good with how we look, we actually feel able to take on the world and all that it throws at us.

Beyond appearances my faith has provided me with a source of strength that has enabled me to cope with things I never believed I could. And I have wonderful friends and family who have been relentless in supporting me through the challenges of the last 12 months.

It has been a long journey and I'm so grateful for not having to make it alone.

66

Mastectomy—A Bloke's Perspective

A few weeks ago I met up with the PR team from Breakthrough Breast Cancer who are going to help me promote this book when it comes out next year. What struck me about the meeting was that the main interest in my story from their perspective is that they recognise there is very little information available to support men who are trying to help wives or partners through a battle with breast cancer. In some, small, tiny way they think this book may help to fill that void and that is why they are keen to help support the book launch.

So it is with that in mind, and with the need to help me process what we have been through over the past year, that I embark on this post and try to cobble together some coherent thoughts on what it has been like to be a husband watching his wife go through a cancer battle and a mastectomy. And I want to make clear from the start that I do this in the context that the difficulties I have faced over the last twelve months pale into insignificance compared to what Miranda has been through. And that is why I wanted this post to follow Miranda's story. It is without doubt, a much better place to be the bystander than the individual engaged in the battle. But it is still not easy or pleasant and having experienced it; this is what I now know.

So where do I start? Well, let's be honest, for a bloke, your wife's breasts are a major part of the more intimate and physical side of your relationship. When Miranda was diagnosed there was the initial shock and obvious, natural concern for her welfare, both in the short and long term. I think I went through a process of just trying to get my head around the news and how we were going to cope. And then inevitably, the thought turns to what impact this would all have on me. I still haven't decided whether this is because I have a deep lying tendency to be selfish or whether that is just a natural reaction that most men would have.

At the outset there was some debate about whether she would need a lumpectomy (removal of just part of the breast) or a full mastectomy. There was even some suggestion that maybe a double mastectomy would be advisable. I can remember vividly thinking that Miranda had to have whatever was going to give her the best hope of surviving and that I would be vehement in supporting her, irrespective of what that operation might be. Secretly I'll admit to hoping desperately that this would turn out to be just a lumpectomy!

As you now know it transpired that Miranda was going to need a mastectomy and I was careful not to try to influence her decision but grateful too that she was determined to go for an immediate reconstruction. I had a fear about how a one-sided wife would affect the physical side of our relationship.

And whilst I find myself talking about the "ahem" (coughs nervously) physical side of our relationship let me set the context into which this concern was being considered in my head. One of the side effects of the chemotherapy that Miranda was undergoing was the suppressing of her libido. Our relationship went from being one with a normal physical aspect to it, to one that was largely platonic. And I want to point this out because it took a fortuitous bit of internet research on my part to discover this consequence of her type of chemotherapy. We had lots of leaflets and explanations but no one told us about this particular side effect and I think, as a bloke, this would have been a good thing to have been told in advance.

The best way I can describe the impact of a cancer diagnosis on a relationship is that it is like being caught in a whirlwind. There is so much to cope with, so many changes, so much worry and everything feels under threat. Dealing with your partner rejecting any attempt at intimacy would have been easier to deal with if the reason why they did so was understood. One less perceived threat to deal with.

As the story transpired Miranda had her mastectomy in the summer but was denied an immediate reconstruction due to her low blood count and now, where once was her right breast, is a large red scar. But to be totally honest that has been so much easier to get used to then I ever expected. And that has caused me to re-evaluate what is at the root of a relationship, what is at the heart of attraction. What really is love all about?

Those questions have made me go back and watch a "Nooma" DVD produced by Rob Bell which explores what it really means to love someone as we were created to. In it he looks at three Hebrew words which all translate to mean love.

I do think that sometimes we struggle to express what we really feel, not because we haven't the capability to describe it but simply because the English language doesn't allow us too. Take the word "love". We use it in so many different contexts. I love going to Starbucks and I love my wife.

One word. Two very different meanings.

In Hebrew there is a word for love which is "raya". Raya would translate as the love you have for a friend, your mates.

I have raya love for the people I work with, for my cricket mates, for the people I hang out with, my business partner and "bestie" Steve and, of course, I have raya love for Miranda too. We met through work and our relationship was purely a raya love kind of relationship before it developed into something more.

The second Hebrew word for love is "ahava". This is a far deeper love, far more profound than a fleeting romantic feeling. It is about being totally commited to another person. It is knowing that you just want to be with them. Ahava love means that you feel a little bit lost when you are not with that person. I have ahava love for Miranda.

Finally there is the "dode" love in Hebrew which literally translates as "to fondle." This is the lust part of love, the physical element. And I suppose the thought at the back of any blokes mind (and mine) is that when their wife goes through an operation, like a mastectomy, that will change her physical appearance, is will this affect my dode?!

What the Rob Bell DVD reminded me was that we are created to be in a relationship with someone for which we have all of the above three types of love. He creates the analogy of each of them as flames and that we need all three flames burning and entwined. We are never going to be completely satisfied without having all those three flames burning.

You see when we are younger there is a real temptation to focus on the dode type of love. We get into relationships, or at least I did, where the dode flame burns really hot for a while but because we have no real ahava love for the other person the flame goes out and the relationship ends. In my experience, that can be a painful and unfulfilling process to go through.

So I think what I've learnt as a bloke with a wife going through breast cancer is this.

Cancer will test your relationship, challenge it, and maybe even threaten it a little. But if you are going through it with someone for whom you have the deepest raya love and a real sense of ahava then cancer cannot break it.

And what about the dode?

Does the change in physical appearance affect the physical relationship?

Well I've learnt that when you have all three flames burning, when your ahava is on fire, then dode burns as strongly as it ever did. The heat of the love is way too powerful to worry about the disappearance of some fatty tissue in the chest area.

Especially when that tissue contained a poisonous lump that threatened the life of the person that you know deep down you were created to be with.

67

A Different Way

I love Christmas. I love everything about it. I love the atmosphere in the shops in the build up. I love the carols and the songs. Well OK maybe there are only so many times that you can listen to Roy Wood's "I wish it could be Christmas everyday" but you get my point. And I love mince pies and mulled wine. I love decorating the tree. I love turkey, cranberry sauce and Christmas pudding with brandy butter. Do you know I can even cope with brussel sprouts! I love the excuse to have a whisky that has been "left out for Father Christmas." I love playing board games around the fire. I love the anticipation of Christmas. I love buying presents and I love the excitement of opening them on Christmas day too.

But most of all I love the reason why we celebrate Christmas. I love the Christmas story. I love the sense of wonder that it evokes. I love the fact that a God so awesome and powerful should make himself human in such a vulnerable way and in such a humble setting. And I love the sense of the promise fulfilled. I love the fact that we have a God who loves us so much that He came to be with us, experience all the emotions that we do as we live out our lives.

Now isn't it funny when you think you know every element of a story and then suddenly something pops out at you that you had never noticed before. Well I was listening to the Christmas story earlier this month and one line has resonated with me like it never has before. It's the bit where the three wise men have presented their gifts and are about to leave. There are just three words I'd never noticed before. It's at the end of the sentence that says something to the effect that the three wise men then left and went home . . . . a different way.

Of course this could just mean that they left for home and took the Bethlehem by-pass rather than risk going through the town centre. Indeed they probably did take a different route as they were fairly keen to avoid old King Herod on their way. But I was listening to a talk by one of my favourite authors, Max Lucado, who was considering whether perhaps the three wise men actually left that meeting and went on to behave and live their lives in a different way as a result of what they had experienced. I think if I had been there and witnessed God in a manger, the impact would have been so profound that I would have left and gone on to live my life in a different way.

If you have been following this blog for a while you will know that I'm captivated by stories. I've realised that as we all live out our lives, we tell a story. And I've realised that it is completely down to us as to how good the story is that we tell. We can't necessarily control the scenes and the environment in which our story is set, but we can control how we deal with the situations in which we find ourselves. We write the storyline.

The three wise men followed a star and ended up meeting God in person. They could have carried on living their lives telling the same story but they chose to go home a different way.

That all sounds blindingly obvious really but I was reminded that when we are faced with dramatic scenes or life changing moments in our lives we don't always change the story we are telling. On a long drive home this week I was listening to a radio programme about homelessness. It was a tough programme to listen to but one of the things talked about is that Christmas is the time of year when most homeless people are rehoused as there is a concerted effort by government agencies and charities to get people off the streets. According to the programme around an amazing 75% of those homeless people who are found permanent homes at Christmas will be back on the streets by the end of March. It struck me that we generally don't do change very well. Sometimes, just like those homeless people, we are telling a story that isn't that attractive but we don't always take the chances to change the story because we are so familiar with it. So, no matter how bad the story, it is one we are comfortable with, and so we just keep telling it. We don't take the opportunity to travel on in a different way.

A year ago today I started this blog. I wrote the very first entry whilst sat with my wife as she had her very first dose of chemotherapy having just been diagnosed with breast cancer. One year on I am writing the final entry in totally different circumstances, at home and with Miranda's cancer gone, hopefully forever. Of course, Miranda still has some more Herceptin treatment to go through and the not insignificant issue of reconstructive surgery but this feels a good place to close this chapter of our story. This is the final entry in The Last Chocolate Brownie.

Thank you so much for walking this journey with us. Your support, messages, comments and encouragement has been invaluable to us along the way.

The one question I have been asked more than any other over the last few weeks is this. Do I think the experience of Miranda's battle with cancer has changed me? I always think that self analysis is so difficult but I am currently thinking that it hasn't. I don't think I am a different person for the experience.

Obviously I never chose that cancer battle scene in which to live out our story for a while. And parts of the story have been brutal, difficult and uncomfortable. But parts of the story have also been amazingly encouraging, empowering and enthralling. And the overriding feeling is that I have learnt so much. I have discovered things about myself and my family over the past year that without living through this experience I would never have learnt.

And I am determined to move on in a different way. I am determined to make my story as compelling and exciting as I can. And I want to be the kind of husband and Dad that encourages my wife and children to do the same.

We are all on a once in a lifetime journey. Literally. We can't always influence the twists and turns that we will face but we can totally control the manner in which we take them.

Thank you for reading our story.

If I have one wish to leave you with, it is this.

My wish is that by travelling with us, by reading our story, you may in some small, tiny way have been encouraged to live just the best story you can.

And, if that means you need to continue your journey in a different way, may you find the courage to do so.

Travel well.

Printed in Great Britain
by Amazon.co.uk, Ltd.,
Marston Gate.